WORKBOOK TO ACCOMPANY CONQUER MEDICAL CODING

A Critical Thinking Approach
with Coding Simulations
2018

MEDICAL CODING

WORKBOOK TO ACCOMPANY

CONQUER MEDICAL CODING

2018

A Critical Thinking Approach with Coding Simulations

Jean H. Jurek, MS, RHIA
President
Jean Jurek Associates Inc., Medical Coding Solutions Company
Clarence, NY

Stacey Mosay, RHIA, CCS-P, COC
Policy Solutions Manager
Cotiviti Healthcare, Atlanta, GA
Consultant
Private Practice Solutions, Charleston, SC

Daphne Neris, CPC, CCS-P, CPC-I
Consultant
Branford, CT

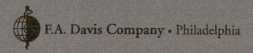

F.A. Davis Company • Philadelphia

F.A. Davis Company
1915 Arch Street
Philadelphia, PA 19103
www.fadavis.com

Last digit indicates print number: 10 9 8 7 6 5 4 3 2 1

Publisher, Health Professions: Quincy McDonald
Director of Content Development, Health Professions: George W. Lang
Senior Developmental Editor, Health Professions: Dean W. DeChambeau
Manager of Design and Illustration: Carolyn O'Brien

Current Procedural Terminology (CPT) is copyright © 2017 American Medical Association. All Rights Reserved. No fee schedules, basic units, relative values, or related listings are included in CPT. The AMA assumes no liability for the data contained herein. Applicable FARS/DFARS restrictions apply to government use. CPT® is a trademark of the American Medical Association.

As new scientific information becomes available through basic and clinical research, recommended treatments and drug therapies undergo changes. The author and publisher have done everything possible to make this book accurate, up-to-date, and in accord with accepted standards at the time of publication. The author, editors, and publisher are not responsible for errors or omissions or for consequences from application of the book, and make no warranty, expressed or implied, in regard to the contents of the book. Any practice described in this book should be applied by the reader in accordance with professional standards of care used in regard to the unique circumstances that may apply in each situation. The reader is advised always to check product information (package inserts) for changes and new information regarding dose and contraindications before administering any drug. Caution is especially urged when using new or infrequently ordered drugs.

ISBN-13: 978-0-8036-6940-6

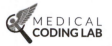 Conquer the type of complex coding scenarios you will face every day in your career by accessing **Medicalcodinglab.com**. Medical Coding Lab is an online interactive program featuring interactive capstone cases, documentation analysis exercises, and code building challenges with feedback. F.A. Davis Company created Medical Coding Lab specifically for *Conquer Medical Coding*. Every activity corresponds with the content in the text. Use the access code printed in the front of your text and begin developing the investigative skills you will need for a successful career in medical coding.

Contents

CHAPTER 1

Your Career as a Medical Coder

When health-care providers examine or treat patients, they use clinical terms to document the patients' medical diagnoses and procedures in medical records. To be able to analyze and track how these conditions are treated and to bill for the medical services, medical codes must be assigned to the narrative clinical text. Knowledgeable medical coders help ensure the maximum appropriate payment for medical services. Successful completion of this program is your first step on the path to a rewarding career as a medical coder. Chapter 1 in *Conquer Medical Coding* describes and explains:

- The purposes of medical coding
- The concept of medical necessity and the way that medical coding links diagnoses and procedures to establish it
- The types of health-care organizations that employ medical coders
- The relationship between documentation, coding, and billing
- The basic steps in the medical coding process
- The skills, attributes, and behaviors that successful medical coders exemplify
- The opportunities for professional certification as a medical coder

MULTIPLE CHOICE

Select the option that best completes the statement or answers the question.

1. Which of the following is not an AHIMA certification?
   A. CCS-P
   B. COC
   C. RHIA
   D. RHIT

2. Health-care expenses amount to 3.46 trillion dollars. Of that amount, 2.8 trillion represents which of the following expenses (select three)?
   A. Nutritional supplements
   B. Professional services
   C. Prescription drugs
   D. Hospital care

3. Which of the following agencies are not part of the government-sponsored health-care programs?
   A. Medicare
   B. Kaiser Permanente
   C. Medicaid
   D. CHAMPVA

4. Which of the following is not a front office duty (select two)?
   A. Scheduling
   B. Billing
   C. Registration
   D. Collections

5. In the hospital's charge entry system, what document provides input for services the patient has received?
   A. Charge slip
   B. Encounter form
   C. CDM
   D. Practice Management Program

6. Medical coders can find employment in both traditional and nontraditional settings. Which of the following is a nontraditional setting?
   A. Hospital
   B. Insurance company
   C. Physician practice
   D. Outpatient clinic

7. A hospital has an opening in their medical records department for a certified coder who can examine medical records for accuracy to help with information for medical research and statistical data. Which of the following is the correct certification for this position?
   A. CPC
   B. CCS
   C. CCS-P
   D. RHIT

8. Under AHIMA's code of ethics, a health information management professional shall not:
   A. Consult with a colleague in taking remedial action for a colleague's incompetence or impairment
   B. Hide or ignore review outcomes, such as performance data
   C. Take measures to discourage unethical conduct of colleagues
   D. Be knowledgeable about policies and procedures

9. In the third step of the medical coding process, the medical coder will abstract (select three):
   A. Diagnoses
   B. Procedures
   C. Patient's health insurance
   D. Other conditions that affect treatment

10. An applicant for a coding position arrived late for her interview. How should the applicant handle this situation?
    A. Explain that she had car trouble so it isn't her fault
    B. Apologize and indicate that this was an unusual occurrence for her
    C. Indicate that being late was never a problem at her previous job
    D. Explain that with three children it is difficult to get everyone out of the house on time

SHORT ANSWER

Answer the following questions.

1. A form that contains a summary of the provider's services is referred to in two ways. What are they?

   _____

2. Are patients seen in the hospital's emergency department (ED) considered outpatient or inpatient?

   _____

   _____

3. A patient's explanation of the reason why he or she is being seen is what part of SOAP?

   _____

4. The patient's primary illness, symptoms, or other treated conditions are designated as:

   _____

5. The book that contains symptoms, illnesses, and so on, is referred to as:

   _____

   _____

6. What is the code set used by inpatient facilities for procedure codes?

   _____

   _____

7. Health plans set up by employers to cover medical services for employees are referred to as:

   _____

8. A coder sent a job application to the administrative department of a local hospital. The application was returned with an explanation that there is a more appropriate department for her coding skills. Which department is that?

   _____

   _____

9. Hospitals compete with physician practices for outpatient services by setting up what two types of outpatient facilities?

   _____

   _____

10. What document might a physician provide when accused of not treating a patient correctly?

   _____

11. A coder in a physician practice wants to advance in her career and decides to become certified. She is confused by how many certifications are available. Which coding certification would be the most appropriate?

_____

_____

12. The CDM is an appropriate system for which health-care environment?

_____

_____

13. "Be knowledgeable about established policies and procedures for handling concerns about colleagues' unethical behavior" is part of which coding certification agency's code of ethics?

_____

14. What federal law requires hospital EDs to treat patients regardless of their ability to pay?

_____

15. What is the process that efficiently translates long descriptions of physician services so that they can be universally understood?

_____

_____

16. What set of codes describes procedures performed in the inpatient hospital setting?

_____

17. Medical coding is part of a process that bridges between clinical data and the billing process that generates payment for medical services. What is that process called?

_____

_____

18. Which payer is a 100% federally funded health plan?

_____

_____

19. Medical coders are able to work in several environments. Name one other than the physician's office or hospital.

_____

_____

20. Because of the advances in medical technology, many medical services are provided in the outpatient setting instead of the inpatient setting. Name one of those services.

_____

_____

CASE STUDIES

1. Brenda S.

   A local hospital ED has been inundated with influenza patients because of the lack of immunizations in their area. Brenda, the admitting nurse, finds that over 70% of the patients have no insurance and has asked for guidance regarding how this should be handled. The ED supervisor indicates that there is a law that requires hospital EDs to treat patients regardless of their ability to pay.

   Is the supervisor correct and, if so, what is that law?

   _____

   _____

2. Kaylah M.

   During an interview for a job as a medical coder, Kaylah, the applicant, was asked about her communication skills. Kaylah replied that she didn't need communication skills because she works with documents and computers and doesn't need to communicate with anyone.

   Is the applicant correct and is she likely to be hired? Explain your answer.

   _____

   _____

3. George M.

   After working for 15 years in an internal medicine office, George, an experienced coder, applies for a job at a medical school to work as a coder for their internal medicine clinic. When asked about a coding certification, George explains that, after working for 15 years in the coding field, a certification wasn't necessary, because he knew everything he needed to know.

   Is the applicant correct? Explain your answer.

   _____

   _____

4. JoAnn D.

   JoAnn was seen in a dermatologist's office because she wanted to remove a blemish on her arm. The dermatologist carefully examined the blemish and assured the patient that it was not a malignancy and would cause her no harm. The blemish had been there many years and the patient was nervous about it and wanted it removed.

   Is the removal medically necessary and would it be covered by her health insurance?

   _____

   _____

5. Amelia C.

   Amelia, the wife of a veteran, is seen in a physician's office for asthma. Her insurance is CHAMPVA and is under her husband's name. The coder explains that CHAMPVA covers only the veteran, not the family, and the patient is responsible for the physician's fee.

   Is the coder correct? Explain what coverage CHAMPVA provides.

   _____

   _____

6. Bob C.

Bob, a 60-year-old male patient, presents to his primary physician for ingrown toenails on his right foot. The physician treats the toenails by trimming them and instructs the patient to soak them and change his footwear. If Bob does not follow this regimen, he will need surgery to remove the toenails.

What abnormal condition is the patient being treated for and what instructions was the patient given?

_____

_____

7. Kim L.

Kim, a 70-year-old patient, goes to the ED with chest pain. Her medical history shows hypertension and diabetes with coronary artery disease. She has had several surgeries over the years related to her coronary artery disease. There is concern that Kim is still getting chest pain. She is given nitroglycerin, which relieves the chest pain, but is instructed to see her cardiologist as soon as possible.

Was the patient given treatment for her symptom and what further instruction was provided?

_____

_____

8. Alvin O.

Alvin is seen in the dermatologist's office for warts on the right big toe and the left heel. He has tried to treat this problem himself by trimming them but they keep returning and are increased in size. He asks that they be removed. After his examination of Alvin, the dermatologist uses a CO_2 laser to vaporize both warts.

What condition did the patient present with and what treatment was given?

_____

_____

9. Kent M.

Kent, a coder, has applied for a position at a large physician practice after working for many years in the hospital. In the interviewer's notes, she indicates that Kent was dressed in jeans and a tee shirt and was late for the appointment. Kent explained that this was how he dressed at the hospital and there was a lot of traffic that day.

Would the physician practice hire this coder? Explain your answer?

_____

_____

10. Sandy K.

In an interview at a gastroenterology practice, Sandy, a coder, indicated that she had over 30 years of experience in billing and coding. When she started at her former job, patients were billed on green billing cards that she filled out after each patient encounter, copied, and then mailed to the patients. Patients were responsible for the bill and they had to apply to their insurance company for reimbursement. Sandy felt that all this computer billing was making more work for billers and coders.

Is the coder describing a coding position or a billing position? Would she be hired?

_____

_____

INTERNET RESEARCH

1. The Internet is a valuable source of information about many topics of interest to medical coders. For example, to explore career opportunities, study the job statistics gathered by the *Occupational Outlook Handbook* of the Bureau of Labor Statistics at http://stats.bls.gov/oco. Using the search tool, enter a job title of interest, such as health information technician. In particular, review the job outlook information.
2. Visit www.alliedhealthcareers.com, and use the search feature to research positions available in the category of Health Information Management/Medical Records. List five job titles that you find in the coding area.

M E D I C A L **CODING LAB** Remember to use the coding activities at **Medicalcodinglab.com** for extra practice on what you have just learned and to test your knowledge.

The Regulatory Environment of Coding

Chapter 2 in *Conquer Medical Coding* introduces the laws and regulations that apply to coding by explaining the types of documentation with which coders work. It is the patients' medical records—containing the chronological and comprehensive documentation of their health history and status—that providers use to communicate and coordinate health care and that serve as the basis for medical coding. Chapter 2 also describes and explains:

- The importance of the documentation in medical records to the medical coding process
- The requirements for, and procedures used to guard the confidentiality of patients' protected health information under the HIPAA Privacy Rule
- The purpose of the HIPAA Security Rule and the Breach Notification Rule
- The required disease, procedure, and supply code sets under the HIPAA Electronic Health Care Transactions and Code Sets standards
- Fraud and abuse in health care
- The use of compliance plans to ensure accurate and compliant medical coding

MULTIPLE CHOICE

Select the option that best completes the statement or answers the question.

1. A history and examination (H&P) requires which of the following (select three)?
   A. Chief complaint
   B. Diagnosis and assessment
   C. Treatment plan
   D. The individual responsible for the bill

2. A compliance officer or committee authority has many responsibilities. Select the answer that is not one of those responsibilities.
   A. Review collected data
   B. Fire employees not in compliance
   C. Interview employees
   D. Report potential fraud, waste, and abuse within the organization

3. To prepare the type of document referred to as de-identified health information requires which of the following?

A. Names must be removed

B. Medical record numbers must be removed

C. The patient's diagnosis must be removed

D. Health plan beneficiary numbers must be removed

4. In an evaluation and management (E/M) encounter/visit, the patient's history has several elements. Which of the following are examples of those elements (select three)?

A. History of present illness

B. Examination

C. Review of systems

D. Past medical history

5. Immediate access to health information, computerized physician order management, automated alerts, and reminders are examples of the advantages of which of the following documents?

A. Operative report

B. Discharge summary

C. Electronic health record

D. E/M service

6. Privacy Rule, Security Rule, and Electronic Health Care Transactions and Code Sets standards are part of what law enacted in 1996?

A. HIPAA

B. CPT

C. ICD-10

D. The Affordable Health Care Act

7. Under HIPAA, TPO represents:

A. Transfer, provider, order

B. Treatment, payment, health-care operations

C. Treatment, provider, health-care orders

D. Transfer, payment, health-care operations

8. Select the answer that does not apply under the Monitoring and Auditing Work Plans section of a compliance plan.

A. Include a process for responding to results

B. Identify a time limit for closing an investigation

C. Outline monitoring/auditing specifics

D. Include corrective actions

9. There are exceptions to the minimum necessary standard under HIPAA. Which of the following is not one of those exceptions?

A. Statutory reports

B. Workers' compensation cases

C. Informed consent for surgery

D. Court orders

10. Select the answer that does not meet the criteria for an E/M encounter.

A. An encounter to perform surgery

B. An encounter about the patient's current complaint

C. An encounter to determine if surgery is needed

D. A hospital postoperative visit

SHORT ANSWER

Answer the following questions.

1. The patient's reason for the visit is often referred to as the chief complaint. What is the other term used to describe the chief complaint?

_____

_____

2. When a patient is scheduled for surgery, the physician discusses assessment, risks, and recommendations and asks the patient to sign a document. What is the document called?

_____

_____

3. During a patient's final hospital visit with his or her physician, the physician will document the discussion regarding the patient's final diagnosis, current condition, and prognosis, and give instructions for any special needs or restrictions. This documentation is referred to as the:

_____

_____

4. Organizing a patient's health record in chronological order using a systematic, logical, and consistent method is considered:

_____

_____

5. What specific office of the federal government enforces health-care fraud and abuse laws?

_____

_____

6. Is intentionally coding for services that were not performed considered fraud or considered abuse?

_____

_____

7. After visiting with her cousin, a patient comes into the clinic because she found out that her cousin has tuberculosis. The patient is worried that she has the same illness, although she does not show any signs or symptoms of that illness. The coder reports a diagnosis of tuberculosis. Is the coder correct?

_____

_____

8. "Young adults up to age 26 can remain as dependents on their parents' private health insurance plan" is an element of what federal law enacted in 2010?

_____

_____

9. Under HIPAA, the electronic data that is regularly sent between providers, health plans, and employers is referred to as:

_____

_____

10. The main federal government agency responsible for health-care regulation is:

_____

_____

11. The Joint Commission was formerly named:

_____

_____

12. Before the Affordable Health Care Act, payers were allowed to drop a beneficiary from a plan because of a preexisting condition. This practice was known as:

_____

_____

13. Because each CPT code has its own separate fee, are coders allowed to code all services separately?

_____

_____

14. The organization that works with the U.S. Department of Justice, including the Federal Bureau of Investigation, to prosecute medical fraud and abuse is:

_____

_____

15. Name the two parts of compliance plans that are most important to coders.

_____

_____

16. Must the patient's chief complaint always be documented in clinical terms?

_____

_____

17. The interpretation of information obtained in an E/M service is the:

_____

_____

18. Documenting a patient's progress and response to a treatment plan is referred to as:

_____

_____

19. Information provided by medical coders can lead to additional financial reward for physicians by following the best medical practices to ensure a patient's health; this is referred to as:

_____

_____

20. Medical credentials are among the criteria required for physicians by payers in order to meet a payer's professional standards. What is another criteria?

_____

_____

CASE STUDIES

1. Stella V.

   An employee of a nationwide insurance company has interviewed an applicant who sees Dr. Olson. The employee knows Stella, who is a coder at Dr. Olson's office, and calls her to ask about any medical problems the applicant has. Stella goes through the applicant's record and indicates what diagnoses the applicant has.

   Is it appropriate for the coder to reveal this information to a prospective employer? Explain your answer.

   _____

   _____

2. Tanya G.

   Tanya, a 3-year-old patient, presented to her pediatrician with an earache and abdominal pain. The physician treated Tanya and prescribed an antibiotic and clear liquids for gastroenteritis. Tanya's mother then asked to speak to the office manager regarding a problem. She explained that she had recently changed health-care carriers and that the new coverage wouldn't be valid until the next week. The mother asked that the office just change the date of the visit so that she could be covered for the physician's charges.

   Should the office manager comply with the mother's request? Explain your answer.

   _____

   _____

3. Bai Z.

   Bai, a 51-year-old male, has a history of aortic valve replacement, pacemaker/defibrillator insertion, bradycardia, and cardiomyopathy. He is at the emergency department (ED) because he has had bilateral lower extremity swelling for 5 days with shortness of breath. Bai does not follow a cardiac diet of any kind and does not exercise. He states that it is too difficult for him to walk. He has not seen a cardiologist or primary care physician in over a year and now presents to the ED. After examination, chest x-ray, and laboratory studies, the physician determines Bai has congestive heart failure and will need to increase his Lasix dosage. He must see both his primary care physician and cardiologist as soon as possible.

   Identify the patient's symptoms.

   _____

   _____

4. Mia F.

   Mia was diagnosed with a nasal tumor. The nose was injected with a solution of 1% Xylocaine with epinephrine through an intercartilaginous route. A right intercartilaginous incision was made and the entire nasal dorsum was exteriorized. A full firm tumor approximately 1 to 2 cm in diameter was located on the lateral nasal bone. The surgeon separated the tumor from the skin and from below. The tumor was removed and sent for pathology.

What procedure was performed and what diagnostic services were also indicated?

_____

_____

5. Elisa D.

Two of the front desk personnel who have worked together for several years in a large orthopedic practice have become close friends. While reviewing the patient folders for today's schedule, Elisa discovers that her neighbor is coming in to see one of the physicians later today. Elisa discusses her neighbor's condition with her friend while signing patients in at the front desk for their visits.

Is this a HIPAA violation and, if so, which type is this?

_____

_____

6. Betty N.

After passing her CPC proficiency examination, the newest coder in the orthopaedic practice began using HCPCS Q codes to identify cast supplies provided to patients. As the insurance carrier's denials came through, Betty realized that the Q codes were being denied on all the claims she coded. She contacted the health insurance company and asked why they were denying HCPCS codes. The reply was that they don't have HCPCS codes in their system, they don't use them, and she should find a different code.

Is the insurance company correct? Explain your answer.

_____

_____

7. Max C.

On the day Max left the hospital, the attending physician asked him questions and provided information such as Max's final diagnosis, information on his current condition, and the results from any x-rays and/or laboratory results. The physician indicated a hospital visit on the medical record but the coder felt it was discharge day management.

Who is correct and why?

_____

_____

8. Wendy A.

Wendy, a patient, has been having problems with headaches and an abnormal gait for many years. Following her last appointment, her physician refers her to a neurologist to determine if she may have early onset of Parkinson's disease. The encounter form is filled out and the physician writes "? Parkinson's" on the form. The coder uses the diagnosis code for Parkinson's disease.

Is the coder correct? Explain your answer.

_____

_____

9. Ephram S.

The following information was dictated as part of the physician's evaluation of Ephram: Head is normal. Ears are clear. Eyes are clear. Pupils are equal, round, and reactive to light and accommodation. Throat is clear. Nose is clear. Neck has good range of motion without nodes. Lungs are clear. Heart has regular heart rate and rhythm. Abdomen is soft without masses. Testicles are descended. Back is straight. He is walking well. He has good muscle tone. See developmental forms in chart.

This documentation represents what part of an E/M service?

_____

_____

10. EHR Advantage

"The EHR is simultaneously accessible to all qualified users. Compared to sorting through papers in a paper folder, an EHR database can save time when vital patient information is needed. Once information is updated in a patient record, it is available to all who need access, whether across the hall or across town."

This information represents which advantage of an electronic health record?

_____

_____

INTERNET RESEARCH

Review the information on enforcement of the Privacy Rule on the website of the federal government's Office for Civil Rights.

MEDICAL CODING LAB Remember to use the coding activities at **Medicalcodinglab.com** for extra practice on what you have just learned and to test your knowledge.

CHAPTER 3

ICD-10-CM Basics

The *International Classification of Diseases, Tenth Revision, Clinical Modification* (ICD-10-CM) code set is a classification system for converting medical diagnoses into numbers. The ICD-10-CM, which replaces the ICD-9-CM code set, contains more than 2,000 categories of disease, many more than the ICD-9-CM. These expanded categories create more codes to permit more specific reporting of diseases and newly recognized conditions. Providers can communicate with payers such as Medicare and insurance companies about the reason for services (the diagnoses) by using these precise standardized codes.

Chapter 3 in *Conquer Medical Coding* introduces the format of the ICD-10-CM and the conventions and rules that assist the coder in finding different types of codes. The chapter next explains the basic process of assigning ICD-10-CM diagnosis codes. In addition, Chapter 3 includes the following topics:

- The background and history of ICD-10-CM
- The roles of the NCHS, CMS, AHIMA, and the AHA in maintaining and updating ICD-10-CM codes
- The statistical use of ICD-10-CM coding data
- The *ICD-10-CM Official Guidelines for Coding and Reporting*
- The organization and content of Volumes 1 and 2 of ICD-10-CM
- How to locate the periodic updates to ICD-10-CM codes using the Internet
- The meaning of "coding to the highest level of specificity"
- Common medical resources used to assist in the assignment of accurate ICD-10-CM codes

CODE IT!

Assign all pertinent ICD-10-CM codes to the following diagnoses or conditions.

1. _____ Acute, recurrent, maxillary sinusitis

2. _____ Hypertrophy of the lingual tonsil and adenoids

3. _____ Pneumonia in anthrax

4. _____ Diabetic mononeuropathy with type 2 diabetes mellitus, insulin dependent

5. _____ Nontoxic multinodular goiter

6. _____ Addison's disease

7. _____ Primary malignant female breast cancer—left lower outer quadrant

8. _____ Acute respiratory failure with hypoxia caused by malignant neoplasm of the lower lobe of the right lung

9. _____ Initial encounter for physical child abuse, without specifying whether sexual or physical; the code will be for child maltreatment

10. _____ Displaced closed fracture of the left tibia, initial episode of care

MULTIPLE CHOICE

Select the option that best provides the correct code, completes the statement, or answers the question.

1. Which of the following code(s) are not coded to the highest level of specificity?
   A. I10
   B. E11.621
   C. O47.00
   D. W11

2. Systolic congestive heart failure with hypertension is coded as:
   A. I50.9
   B. I50.9, I11.0
   C. I11.0, I50.20
   D. I10, I50.20

3. Abnormal liver function tests caused by type 1 diabetes mellitus and cholelithiasis. This is coded as:
   A. E10.9, K80.20
   B. R94.5
   C. R94.5, E10.69, K80.20
   D. E10.9, K80.20, R94.5

4. Sore throat is coded as:
   A. J02.8
   B. J02
   C. J02.9
   D. J02.0

5. Spontaneous tension pneumothorax is coded as:
   A. J93.83
   B. J93.11
   C. J93.12
   D. J93.0

6. Encounter for chemotherapy to treat a malignant neoplasm of the throat is coded as:
   A. Z51.11, C14.0
   B. Z51.10, C14.0
   C. C14.0, Z51.11
   D. C14.0, Z51.10

7. Fall from a horse (person hurt was the rider), noncollision, and initial episode of care is coded as:
   A. W19.XXXA, Y93.52
   B. V80.010A, Y93.52
   C. W19.XXXS, V80.018A
   D. Y93.52

8. Morbid obesity with body mass index of 38 in an adult is coded as:
   A. E66.01, Z68.38
   B. E66.2, Z68.38
   C. E66.01
   D. E66.09, Z68.38

9. Secondary osteoarthritis of multiple sites is coded as:
   A. M15.3
   B. M19.93
   C. M15.0
   D. M15.9

10. L4 herniated disc with radiculopathy is coded as:
   A. M51.9
   B. M51.86
   C. M51.26
   D. M51.16

SHORT ANSWER

Answer the following questions.

1. You are the coding supervisor at a major acute care hospital. What resources would you recommend to ensure that the most current ICD-10-CM/PCS codes are in use in your health-care facility? Remember to address issues such as coding resources and computer systems.

2. When is ICD-10-CM/PCS updated?

3. What is the placeholder character used in ICD-10-CM?

4. Can you code directly from the ICD-10-CM Index? Why or why not?

5. Which "excludes note" is interpreted as "not included here"?

6. What does the term "and" mean in ICD-10-CM?

7. In which section of the ICD-10-CM do you find "code first" and "use additional code" notes?

8. What does the seventh character "S" represent when it is used with category S82?

_____

_____

9. Which section of the ICD-10-CM Index to Diseases and Injuries contains main terms such as *earthquake, accident,* or *explosion*?

_____

_____

10. Which legislation mandates the use of ICD-10-CM?

_____

_____

CASE STUDIES

1. Wyatt M.

   Wyatt presents to Dr. Jones's office complaining of swollen neck glands. Dr. Jones does not find any other physical findings but orders laboratory tests. His impression is localized cervical lymphadenopathy.

   a. *What main term would be utilized to code this case?*

   _____

   _____

   b. *Assign the ICD-10-CM code.*

   _____

   _____

2. Richard P.

   Richard presents with urinary frequency and nocturia. The doctor does not detect any abnormal findings but orders an IVP.

   a. *What are the patient's signs and symptoms?*

   _____

   _____

   b. *Assign the ICD-10-CM codes.*

   _____

   _____

3. Mary R.

   Mary complains of heartburn. Her blood pressure is also noted to be elevated. Dr. Doe prescribes Zantac for Mary's heartburn and advises her to come in for weekly blood pressure checks to determine if she has hypertension.

   a. *What main term is used to code the elevated blood pressure?*

   _____

   _____

   b. *Assign the ICD-10-CM codes for both conditions.*

   _____

   _____

4. Mia Z.

Mia presents to Dr. Jones's office with complaints of right lower quadrant abdominal pain; intermittent—duration 1 month. Mia has whitish-clear nonmalodorous vaginal discharge. Pelvic examination—external genitalia appear within normal limits. Vaginal vault has a white discharge present. Diagnosis: Abdominal pain of unknown etiology. Vaginal discharge.

a. *What is the exact location of the abdominal pain?*

_____

_____

b. *Assign the ICD-10-CM codes.*

_____

_____

5. Francisco C.

Francisco was seen in the clinic this morning and found to have MRSA cellulitis of his left foot. The patient is a long-term diabetic, type 1.

a. *Which instructional note is used to code the infectious organism of MRSA?*

_____

_____

b. *Where is this note located?*

_____

_____

c. *Which coding reference would be utilized to provide the meaning of MRSA?*

_____

_____

d. *Assign the ICD-10-CM codes.*

_____

_____

6. Tyrone I.

Tyrone presents with syncope that occurred at church and is admitted to the hospital. Further evaluation by telemetry monitoring show tachycardia-bradycardia syndrome. The physician recommends a dual-chamber pacemaker insertion. On the second hospital day, Tyrone undergoes pacemaker insertion. No complications develop and he is discharged to home to continue medication for chronic back pain. Diagnosis: Tachycardia-bradycardia syndrome, and chronic back pain.

a. *What symptom(s) does the patient have?*

_____

_____

b. *What main term is used to report the tachycardia-bradycardia syndrome?*

_____

_____

c. *Assign the ICD-10-CM codes.*

_____

_____

7. Hachiro L.

Hachiro, a Medicare patient, is seen in the Ambulatory Surgery Center (ASC) for diagnostic and therapeutic left knee arthroscopy. Postoperative diagnoses are: Chondromalacia of the medial femoral condyle, old posterior horn lateral meniscal tear, villonodular synovitis.

a. *Which coding resource would assist the coder regarding the location of the medial femoral condyle?*

_____

_____

b. *What cross reference is used to report the old tear of the meniscus?*

_____

_____

c. *Assign the ICD-10-CM codes based on surgical findings.*

_____

_____

8. James E.

James is referred to the physician office for consultation on his elevated liver function tests. He is a 37-year-old man with alcohol abuse and hypertension. Laboratory results indicate elevated liver function and normal blood pressure. The physician sets up a liver ultrasound and orders a refill of hypertension medication. James is to return in 1 month for follow-up.

a. *Would you report the alcohol abuse and hypertension?*

_____

_____

b. *Assign the ICD-10-CM code(s).*

_____

_____

9. Tyler B.

Tyler, a 4-year-old patient, was seen today by his pediatrician for fever and red lips. Tyler's mother indicates the boy had a sudden high fever 4 days ago, and yesterday his eyes became red and bloodshot; his lips are also red and cracked, and his tongue is red and bumpy. In addition, he has a rash. These symptoms all started during the last 4 days. There is concern that Tyler has Kawasaki's disease, which is associated with coronary artery aneurysms. A complete blood count, urinalysis, and a sedimentation rate are to be done. Based on these results, the pediatrician may need to order additional tests and an echocardiogram.

a. *What is Kawasaki's disease?*

_____

_____

b. *Which reference would a coder use to find the definition?*

_____

_____

c. *Assign the ICD-10-CM code(s).*

_____

_____

10. Enid L.

Enid presents from the nursing home with flank pain, dysuria, fever, and shortness of breath. Further evaluation confirms urinary tract infection and acute CHF caused by underdosing of Lasix (initial care). This patient also has a stage II sacral decubitus ulcer. Enid was treated with IV antibiotics and Lasix for CHF. Discharge diagnoses: Urinary tract infection; Acute on chronic systolic CHF caused by underdosing of Lasix.

a. *Which section of the ICD-10-CM Index is used to code the underdosing of Lasix?*

_____

_____

b. *What does the abbreviation CHF mean?*

_____

_____

c. *Assign the ICD-10-CM code(s).*

_____

_____

INTERNET RESEARCH

1. The Centers for Medicare and Medicaid Services maintains the current list of ICD-10-PCS procedure codes and references to HIPAA-mandated transactions and code sets. Access the CMS website at www.cms.gov, and click on Regulations and Guidelines to find the details of HIPAA legislation for health-care transactions.
2. The National Center for Health Statistics oversees the changes and modifications to ICD-10-CM. The Coordination and Maintenance Committee provides a mechanism for making changes to codes. Locate the meeting minutes of the Coordination and Maintenance Committee at www.cdc.gov/nchs/icd/icd9cm_maintenance.htm to see how this committee addresses applications for code changes and modifications. (*Hint:* See the section titled Submission of Proposals.)
3. ICD-10-CM codes are used for statistical reporting by federal health agencies such as the Centers for Disease Control and Prevention (CDC). Access the CDC website at www.cdc.gov and find one study or survey that includes ICD-10-CM codes. How are the codes used to provide information? For example, access the report listing the 113 selected causes of death using ICD-10-CM codes at www.cdc.gov/nchs/deaths.htm.
4. Understanding the disease process can make ICD-10-CM coding easier. One website that lists a variety of diseases and conditions is WebMD. Access the WebMD website at www.webmd.com, and find information about the causes, signs and symptoms, treatment, and prevention of asthma. For example, ICD-10-CM codes classify the different types of asthma, so knowledge of this information allows the coder to understand coding issues about this disease.
5. Access the Federal Register, Center for Medicare and Medicaid Services, website at https://www.federalregister.gov/index/2013/centers-for-medicare-medicaid-services. Once at the index, enter the search term "ICD-10-CM." Choose one of the articles listed in the search results, which direct you to the printed Federal Register for that topic. Review the Federal Register starting with the table of contents. Summarize the topic chosen to include the purpose of that legislation. Reference the *Federal Register* publication and page numbers. How would this legislation impact ICD-10-CM coding?

MEDICAL CODING LAB Remember to use the coding activities at **Medicalcodinglab.com** for extra practice on what you have just learned and to test your knowledge.

ICD-10-CM Coding Guidelines

Chapter 4 in *Conquer Medical Coding* explains the basic coding guidelines found in Sections IB, II, III, and IV of the *ICD-10-CM Official Guidelines for Coding and Reporting*. Understanding these guidelines is essential in assigning accurate ICD-10-CM codes and sequencing them correctly. The official guidelines also assist the coder with decisions regarding coexisting conditions, medical history, or medical status that should be reported. Chapter 4 explains when to assign multiple codes for a single condition and when to assign combination codes to reflect multiple conditions. The authors cover the rules on coding both acute and chronic conditions, sequelae (late effects), and conditions that are impending or threatened. All of these factors enable the coder to code to the highest level of specificity. The chapter also covers the following topics:

- The content and source of ICD-10-CM "General Coding Guidelines"
- The coding of conditions that are an integral part of the disease process
- The coding of conditions that are not an integral part of the disease process
- The difference between coding guidelines for multiple codes and combination codes
- The patient care flow and associated documentation in the inpatient setting
- The importance of the Uniform Hospital Discharge Data Set (UHDDS) and its relationship to diagnostic coding
- The guidelines for selecting the principal diagnosis following admission from an observation unit and outpatient surgery
- The criteria for reporting additional diagnoses

CODE IT!

Assign all pertinent ICD-10-CM codes to the following diagnoses or conditions.

1. _____ Unstable angina due to coronary artery disease of the native vessel

2. _____ Hypertensive cardiovascular disease with congestive heart failure

3. _____ Acute cerebral embolism with infarction and resulting spastic hemiplegia

4. _____ Arteriosclerotic ulcer of the left toe and cellulitis of the left foot

5. _____ Initial care for infected vascular bypass graft of the right leg with cellulitis

6. _____ Rheumatoid arthritis with lung involvement; chest x-ray showed incidental finding of osteoarthritis of the spine

7. _____ AIDS with Kaposi's sarcoma of the skin

8. _____ Anaphylactic shock due to accidental bee sting, active care provided

9. _____ Iron deficiency anemia versus acquired hemolytic anemia

10. _____ Acquired coagulation defect. The patient was evaluated for mesenteric lymphadenitis.

MULTIPLE CHOICE

Select the option that best provides the correct code, completes the statement, or answers the question.

1. Which code or codes would be reported for a patient with impending cerebrovascular accident with dysphagia?
   A. I63.9, R13.10
   B. I63.9, R13.19
   C. I69.091
   D. R13.10

2. Which code is not coded to its highest level of specificity?
   A. M54.16
   B. S34.124A
   C. O33.3
   D. I20.9

3. Mary presented with abdominal pain, hematemesis, and dehydration due to an acute gastric ulcer. Which code or codes are reported?
   A. K25.0, E86.0
   B. K25.0, E86.0, R10.9
   C. K25.4, E86.0
   D. K25.4, R10.9

4. Which code is reported for primary malignant neoplasm of the right breast, outer quadrant for a female patient, age 45?
   A. C50.811
   B. C50.711
   C. C50.821
   D. C50.812

5. A patient presented with acute on chronic prostatitis due to pseudomonas and also has dysuria. Which codes are reported?
   A. N41.1, R31.9, B96.5
   B. N41.0, N41.1, B96.5
   C. N41.0, B96.5, R31.9
   D. N41.0, N41.1, B96.5, R31.9

6. The UHDDS definitions are integrated into which legislation?
   A. COBRA laws
   B. TEFRA legislation
   C. UACDS legislation
   D. HIPAA legislation

7. Which of the following statements represents two or more diagnoses that equally meet the definition of principal diagnosis?
   A. Mary is admitted for COPD and heart failure.
   B. Joe is admitted for gallbladder removal; he also has diabetes.
   C. Max presents with hematuria due to renal calculi.
   D. Joan is admitted for thrombosis of her leg graft.

8. Which of the following statements represents a complication of medical care?
   A. Urinary retention
   B. Possible urinary retention
   C. Urinary retention due to prostate surgery
   D. Urinary retention due to prostatic hypertrophy

9. Joe presents to the hospital for treatment of facial cellulitis. Joe has shortness of breath as well. The chest x-ray is positive for atelectasis, and the attending physician documents the diagnoses of facial cellulitis and bronchitis. Which of the following is coded?
   A. Facial cellulitis, bronchitis, atelectasis
   B. Facial cellulitis, atelectasis
   C. Facial cellulitis, bronchitis
   D. Bronchitis and atelectasis

10. Which of the following describes a condition that would have a present on admission indicator of W?
    A. After the second hospital day, the patient shows the physician that he has blood in the urine. He does not know when this started.
    B. After admission, the patient develops a drug rash.
    C. The patient presents with colon cancer and has a known history of hypertension.
    D. The code Z85.3 is assigned.

SHORT ANSWER

Answer the following questions.

1. Write the definition of *principal diagnosis*.

   _____

   _____

2. List the criteria that must be met in order to report a diagnosis or condition as secondary.

   _____

   _____

3. Explain the circumstances in which the present on admission indicator would be N.

   _____

   _____

4. What is the payment unit used for Medicare hospital inpatients?

   _____

   _____

5. If a patient is admitted from outpatient surgery due to a complication, what is the principal diagnosis?

   _____

   _____

6. Which terms identify the presence of comparative or contrasting conditions?

_____

_____

7. Which portion of the medical record contains documentation of the postoperative diagnosis?

_____

_____

8. Terms such as *hospital course* and *final diagnoses* are located in which inpatient report/document in the medical record?

_____

_____

9. When coding an inpatient medical record, the coder should review which document(s) to determine the reason a test was ordered?

_____

_____

10. What is the difference between *rule out* and *ruled out* as they pertain to inpatient coding?

_____

_____

CASE STUDIES

1. Anil S.

    Anil was admitted with impending gangrene of the left lower extremity with diabetic ulcer of the left calf and heel. Anil has known type 2 diabetic peripheral angiopathy and diabetic nephropathy. Discharge diagnosis: Impending gangrene with diabetic peripheral vascular disease and ulcers of the left leg, and diabetic nephropathy.

    a. *Is there a separate code for impending gangrene?*

    _____

    _____

    b. *Assign the ICD-10-CM codes.*

    _____

    _____

2. Alma M.

    Note for Initial Hospital Care

    > **HPI:** Chief complaint is abdominal pain in the mid to lower left quadrant for 2 days. The patient called our office and she was instructed to meet me at the hospital for admission. The pain is sharp and intermittent with a pain scale of 9.
    >
    > **ROS:** The patient denies nausea, vomiting, or diarrhea, no shortness of breath, no dizziness, no musculoskeletal pain, all other systems negative.
    >
    > **PFSH:** History of hypertension and diverticulitis 2 years ago. Her father is currently undergoing treatment for lung cancer. The patient is single and works for the mayor.
    >
    > **MEDS:** Patient takes Procardia.

> **EXAMINATION:** Patient is in distress.
> **VITAL SIGNS:** Temp 101.9, pulse 90, BP 160/99, respiration 22.
> Cardiovascular examination shows regular rate and rhythm, S_1/S_2 normal. The lungs clear to auscultation bilaterally and abdomen is rigid with muted bowel sounds and tender to palpation. Her rectal examination is without stool, no blood is evident. The patient is alert and oriented x3. Her skin is warm and dry, no rashes. Her gait is normal; she has no musculoskeletal pain.
> **MDM:** Diagnosis—Reoccurrence of sigmoid diverticulitis.

a. *Which component of this document supports that there is no associated bleeding?*

_____

_____

b. *Assign the ICD-10-CM code for the principal diagnosis.*

_____

_____

3. Theodore N.

Clinic Note

> **CHIEF COMPLAINT:** Follow-up visit for diabetes and coronary artery disease.
> Fifty-six-year-old male last seen by me 3 months ago. He is taking his medications as directed and has had no hypoglycemic episodes. He denies chest pain, orthopnea, or leg swelling.
> **EXAMINATION:** Appears well and NAD, PB 150/90, weight 210. No jugular vein distention, lungs CTA. Cardiovascular S_1, S_2, no S_3. Abdomen soft, nontender, no masses. Extremities no clubbing or edema, no ulcers.
> **LABS:** Cholesterol 270, HDL 40, LDL 170.
> **MDM:** Diabetes under better control with taking glyburide as directed. Appears compliant. He is to continue glyburide at 10 bid. Continue finger stick. No ischemia but BP still needs work. Increase atenolol to 50 qd. Patient to return in 3 months.

a. *What does the abbreviation HDL mean?*

_____

_____

b. *Assign the ICD-10-CM code(s) for this visit.*

_____

_____

4. Sherman B.

Patient History and Physical Examination

> **PATIENT HISTORY:**
> **CC:** Right arm pain
> Since he woke up this am
> 25-year-old African American male
> Allergic to morphine
> PMH: Sickle-cell anemia
> Takes Lortab and folic acid
> Denies fever, chills, nausea, vomiting, diarrhea, constipation
> No dysuria or pyuria
> Has numbness and tingling in right arm

> **PHYSICAL EXAMINATION:**
> Temp 97, BP 126/85, pulse 95, resp. 16, no acute distress
> HEENT PERRL, conjunctiva pink, turbinates pink, mucous membranes moist
> Neck without lymphadenopathy
> CV S_1, S_2, no edema in extremities
> Resp. CTA bilaterally
> M/S Right arm tender to palpation but does not worsen pain, good range of motion, good strength
> Psychiatric: normal

a. *What is the chief complaint?*

_____

_____

b. *Does the patient have any chronic conditions? If yes, please list.*

_____

_____

c. *Assign the code for history of allergy to morphine. (Hint: Start with the main term "History," sub-term "personal.")*

_____

_____

5. Arron A.

Patient History and Physical Examination

> **PATIENT HISTORY:**
> Patient with suprapubic pain
> Difficulty urinating
> Last urinated 5 hours before coming to hospital
> Now has pain and urge to urinate but cannot
> Denies allergies
>
> **PHYSICAL EXAMINATION:**
> Temp 97, pulse 80, respiration 18, BP 150/90
> HEENT normal
> Chest is clear
> Cardiovascular negative
> Abdomen has suprapubic tenderness and is distended
> **MDM:** Diagnosis-acute urinary retention and prostatism
> 16 French Foley catheter passed with return of 700 cc dark, opalescent urine
> Urinalysis with culture and sensitivity ordered
> If patient continues with voiding problem he is to return to ED
> Patient to follow up in 2 days with his physician
> Meds prescribed
> **DIAGNOSIS:** Acute urinary retention due to enlarged prostate

a. *What are the patient's signs and symptoms?*

_____

_____

b. *Assign the ICD-10-CM code(s).*

_____

_____

6. Sanyoon K.

Patient History and Physical Examination for an Inpatient Hospital Stay

> **PATIENT HISTORY:**
> Nosebleed
> Past medical history of hypertension (HTN), status post cardiac pacemaker insertion, coronary
>   artery disease, medications listed, status post myocardial infarction (MI)
> Nose has bled on and off for 2 weeks
> Today it bled for 30 minutes
> Did not apply pressure, not bleeding now
> Denies chest pain (CP), shortness of breath (SOB), nausea, vomiting, abdominal pain
> No known allergies (NKA)
>
> **PHYSICAL EXAMINATION:**
> General appearance alert, pleasant, no acute distress (NAD)
> Temp 97.5, BP 143/85, pulse 77, respiration 18
> Neck negative
> Nares show dried blood, no active bleeding
> Eyes are clear
> Heart regular rate and rhythm (RRR), no murmurs, no edema in extremities
> Lungs are clear to auscultation (CTA) bilaterally
> Abdomen obese, nontender, soft
> **DIAGNOSIS:** Bilateral epistaxis, resolved, hypertensive heart disease

a. *Does the patient have any diagnoses documented but not listed in the diagnosis list? If yes, please list the additional diagnoses.*

_____

_____

b. *Assign the ICD-10-CM code(s).*

_____

_____

7. Martha D.

Patient History and Physical Examination for an Inpatient Hospital Stay

> **PATIENT HISTORY:**
> Left chest pain
> Right forearm pain
> Nausea
> Past history of migraines, takes Imitrex
> Started while hanging blinds early this afternoon
> 7 of 10 on pain scale
> Pain is constant and radiating
> Pain is worse when moving or breathing
> No attempt made to alleviate pain
> Negative for SOB, emesis, abdominal pain
> Patient is single, does not smoke or drink
>
> **PHYSICAL EXAMINATION:**
> Temp. 98.1, BP 123/87, pulse 83, respiration 100
> Eyes normal
> ENT normal
> Neck normal
> Respiration is CTA bilaterally but positive TTP (tender to palpation) over anterior chest wall
> Cardiac, RRR, no murmurs

> Extremities normal
> GI no tenderness, no masses
> Musculoskeletal normal gait
> Skin cool, dry, good color
> Psych oriented x3, memory normal, mood and affect normal, patient is cooperative with clear speech
> **DIAGNOSIS:** Musculoskeletal chest pain
> **ORDERS:** AP and lateral chest x-ray, EKG, CBC, Qualitative Troponin, pulse oximetry

a. *Has the underlying condition of this patient's pain been determined?*

_____

_____

b. *Assign the ICD-10-CM code(s).*

_____

_____

8. Marion K.

Patient History and Physical Examination for Ambulatory Surgery

> **PATIENT HISTORY:**
> 31-year-old male
> **CC:** Left knee swelling
> Mild edema and erythema
> Pain only when going downstairs
> For 1 week
> Denies fever, chills, nausea, vomiting
> Has been working out on his bike for 4 weeks
> Smokes cigarettes
> Denies any past medical history
> Denies meds
> No known allergies
> **PHYSICAL EXAMINATION:**
> Temp 98, BP 127/77, pulse 64, resp. 18
> M/S left knee painful, TTP, and on flexing
> Skin normal
> Neuro normal
> Psych oriented x3
> **DIAGNOSIS:** Possible acute bursitis of the left knee, aspiration biopsy was completed

a. *What is the outpatient diagnosis that would be reported?*

_____

_____

b. *If this patient was an inpatient, what diagnosis would be reported?*

_____

_____

c. *Assign the ICD-10-CM code(s) for this outpatient visit.*

_____

_____

9. Juanita R.

Juanita presented to the hospital observation unit with shortness of breath, wheezing, and fever. She was observed for moderate persistent asthma with exacerbation. After 28 hours in observation, Juanita's status declined due to acute hypoxic respiratory failure and admission was required.

a. *What is the principal diagnosis for the hospital inpatient stay?*

_____

_____

b. *Assign the ICD-10-CM code(s) for this inpatient.*

_____

_____

10. Rafaele D.

Rafaele presents with elevated amylase and lipase with positive CT scan for acute pancreatitis. He is known to have chronic pancreatitis, which is treated with medication. He has an extensive medical history, which includes alcoholic cirrhosis, history of prostate cancer, and alcohol dependence in remission. The patient was treated with IV fluids, antibiotics, and rest.

Diagnoses: Acute on chronic pancreatitis, cirrhosis, history of prostate cancer, and alcohol dependence (in remission).

a. *Which Official Guideline can be applied to this case regarding the principal diagnosis?*

_____

_____

b. *Assign the ICD-10-CM code(s) for this inpatient.*

_____

_____

INTERNET RESEARCH

1. Locate five medical conditions at the Web MD website at www.webmd.com/a-to-z-guides /common-topics/default.htm. Identify the medical condition and the symptoms that are integral to it. For example, symptoms of asthma include difficulty breathing, wheezing, coughing, and shortness of breath.
2. Knowledge of new technology is essential for keeping up with medical practice and treatment for ICD-10-CM coders. Find a medical website that provides information on the latest technology used to treat heart disease. List the address of the website, and describe the new technology.
3. Research Internet sites that discuss the Uniform Hospital Discharge Data Set. According to your reading, how can coders educate physicians regarding the definition of principal diagnosis and the importance of documentation? See http://health-information.advanceweb.com and the Article Archives at www.fortherecordmag.com/

MEDICAL CODING LAB Remember to use the coding activities at **Medicalcodinglab.com** for extra practice on what you have just learned and to test your knowledge.

CHAPTER 5

ICD-10-CM Chapters 1 Through 5: A00–F99

Correct code assignment and sequencing of patients' diagnosed or suspected conditions are the baseline for gathering data to improve treatment and for demonstrating the medical necessity of procedures. Chapter 5 in *Conquer Medical Coding* describes the steps in selecting codes for infectious diseases, neoplasms, endocrine disorders, illnesses of the blood, and mental illness. In addition, the chapter explains:

- The structure and importance of Section I, Part C of the *ICD-10-CM Official Guidelines for Coding and Reporting*
- The general guideline for selecting and sequencing the causes of infectious diseases
- The major points to consider in code selection and assignment for AIDS/HIV
- The differences among the diagnoses of SIRS and sepsis
- The multiple categories of codes for diabetes mellitus and what distinguishes each category

CODE IT!

Assign all pertinent ICD-10-CM codes to the following diagnoses.

1. _____ Salmonella gastroenteritis

2. _____ Candidiasis infection of the skin (foot)

3. _____ Abscess of the back caused by MRSA

4. _____ Malignant fibrosarcoma of the left tibia with major osseous defect

5. _____ Hb-C sickle-cell crisis with acute chest syndrome

6. _____ Anemia caused by carcinoma of the transverse colon

7. _____ Type 1 diabetic ulcer of great toe, right foot

8. _____ Septic shock caused by *Staphylococcus aureus*

9. _____ 58-year-old with severe protein-energy malnutrition and body mass index (BMI) of 18

10. _____ Sedative dependence with associated sleep disorder and cocaine abuse in remission

MULTIPLE CHOICE

Select the option that best provides the correct code, completes the statement, or answers the question.

1. Metastatic left lower lobe lung cancer is coded as:
   A. C34.32, C79.9
   B. C34.31, C79.9
   C. C78.02, 34.01
   D. C34.32, C80.1

2. Macrocytic anemia secondary to selective vitamin B_{12} malabsorption and proteinuria is coded as:
   A. D51.1
   B. D52.0
   C. D51.1, E52.0
   D. D53.1

3. Acute pancreatitis, alcohol induced in a patient with a cardiac pacemaker insertion 3 years earlier is coded as:
   A. K85.30, T36
   B. K85.20, T34
   C. K85.20, Z95.0
   D. K85.30, Z95.0

4. Female patient with secondary carcinoma of the right lung. She had malignant carcinoma of the thyroid 7 years earlier with no evidence of local recurrence. The codes reported are:
   A. C78.00, Z83.49
   B. C34.90, Z85.850
   C. C34.11, Z83.49
   D. C78.01, Z85.850

5. Herpes simplex caused by HIV infection is coded as:
   A. B20, B00.9
   B. Z11.4, B20
   C. Z11.4
   D. B20, B00.89

6. Pulmonary tuberculosis is coded as:
   A. A15.8
   B. A15.4
   C. A15.5
   D. A15.0

7. Which type of diabetes cannot be treated with oral medications, because these patients do not produce insulin?
   A. Gestational
   B. Type 2
   C. Type 1
   D. Drug-induced

8. The combination of anemia, neutropenia, and thrombocytopenia is coded as:
   A. D64.9, D70.9, D69.6
   B. D61.818
   C. D64.89
   D. D64.8, D70.8, D69.49

9. Poorly controlled diabetes mellitus caused by chronic pancreatitis is coded as:
   A. E08.9, K85.9
   B. E08.9, E08.65, K85.9
   C. E08.65, K86.1
   D. E08.9, K86.1

10. Malignant histiocytoma of the left arm is coded as:
    A. C76.42
    B. C79.89
    C. C49.12
    D. C44.602

SHORT ANSWER

Answer the following questions.

1. Which term in pharmacology refers to the disposition of drugs in the body?

_____

_____

2. What is the generic name for the drug Tamiflu?

_____

_____

3. In ovarian cancer with pelvic lymph node metastasis, what is the primary site of the neoplasm?

_____

_____

4. What are two signs or symptoms associated with sepsis?

_____

_____

5. What is the term used to classify a malignancy that has overlapping sites?

_____

_____

6. A written communication to a physician to clarify documentation of a disease or condition is known as a:

_____

_____

7. How do hematopoietic drugs treat anemia and other cell disorders?

_____

_____

8. Name the type of diabetes that develops during pregnancy.

_____

_____

9. If a person is 5 feet, 5 inches and weighs 245 pounds; his or her weight status is classified as _____ in relationship to BMI.

10. What is the name of the manual used by psychiatrists to report mental disorder terminology?

_____

_____

CASE STUDIES

1. Dolores F.

   Dolores presents with left upper quadrant abdominal pain. Work-up is positive for alcohol-induced acute on chronic pancreatitis. She is alcohol dependent and received counseling.

   a. *Is the symptom of left upper quadrant pain coded?*

   _____

   _____

   b. *Which diagnosis is listed first?*

   _____

   _____

   c. *Code all diagnoses for this case.*

   _____

   _____

2. Johan D.

   Johan is admitted for treatment of a right thoracic mass. The physician performs a right thoracotomy and bronchoscopy. The mass is excised and is determined to be a malignant schwannoma.

   a. *The pathology report would identify the mass as a schwannoma: true or false?*

   _____

   _____

   b. *Code all diagnoses for this case.*

   _____

   _____

3. Akihiro C.

   Akihiro presented with fatigue and low hemoglobin and hematocrit supporting the diagnosis of aplastic anemia. Further evaluation supports that the anemia is caused by chemotherapy. He has received chemotherapy for three sessions to treat his sigmoid colon cancer with liver metastasis.

   a. *What are the documented sign(s) and symptom(s)?*

   _____

   _____

   b. *Which diagnosis is listed first?*

   _____

   _____

   c. *The anemia is an adverse effect of the chemotherapy/antineoplastic drug: true or false?*

   _____

   _____

d. *Code all the diagnoses for this case.*

_____

_____

4. Anisha P.

Anisha presents with fever, leukocytosis, and tachycardia. She has had a urinary tract infection as an outpatient but is not getting better. The diagnosis of *E. coli* sepsis with associated acute renal failure is made and IV antibiotics are started.

a. *Where is the localized infection that is the underlying cause of the systemic infection (sepsis)?*

_____

_____

b. *Should the signs and symptoms of fever, leukocytosis, and tachycardia be coded?*

_____

_____

c. *Does this patient have severe sepsis?*

_____

_____

d. *Code all the diagnoses for this case, listing the primary diagnosis first.*

_____

_____

5. John M.

John is a type 1 diabetic who presents with hypoglycemia caused by an overdose of insulin. The hypoglycemia resulted from a mechanical problem with his insulin pump. John also has diabetic nephropathy and neuropathy.

a. *Is the first-listed diagnosis a complication of the insulin pump?*

_____

_____

b. *Which column from the Table of Drugs and Chemicals is used in this case?*

_____

_____

c. *What are the associated manifestations of his diabetes?*

_____

_____

d. *What condition occurred because of the accidental overdose of insulin?*

_____

_____

e. *Code all the diagnoses for this case, listing the primary diagnosis first.*

_____

_____

6. Walter P.

Walter presents in cocaine withdrawal and alcohol withdrawal with delirium. He also smokes cigarettes. Because of years of alcohol dependence, Walter has alcoholic cirrhosis of the liver. To complicate his care, he also suffers from paranoid schizophrenia.

a. *Can either drug withdrawal or alcohol withdrawal be listed first?*

_____

_____

b. *Code all the diagnoses for this case.*

_____

_____

7. Bridget C.

Bridget presents for her second radiation therapy visit for treatment of her left-sided breast carcinoma located in the left outer quadrant. She is morbidly obese with a BMI of 50.2.

a. *Which section of the ICD-10-CM Official Guidelines provides guidance in sequencing the principal diagnosis for this case?*

_____

_____

b. *What is the first listed diagnosis code?*

_____

_____

c. *Report all other codes for this case.*

_____

_____

8. Jacalyn C.

Jacalyn has dysuria and flank pain. Further evaluation is positive for acute on chronic cystitis. Cultures are positive for MRSA. She also has hypokalemia and hypomagnesemia, which is treated with intravenous fluid additives.

a. *What are the signs and symptoms of the underlying disease?*

_____

_____

b. *What is the organism known as MRSA?*

_____

_____

c. *Should the acute or chronic cystitis be sequenced first?*

_____

_____

d. *Code all the diagnoses for this case, listing the primary diagnosis first.*

_____

_____

9. Benton K.

Benton presents because of gangrene of the left second toe. He is a type 2 insulin-dependent diabetic with known diabetic peripheral vascular disease. After physician query, it is determined that the gangrene is caused by the diabetes.

a. *Code all the diagnoses for this case, listing the primary diagnosis first.*

_____

_____

10. Clayton C.

Clayton has enlarged lymph nodes, weakness, fever, and flu-like symptoms. He is a known IV heroin user. Also noted on chest x-ray is *Pneumocystis carinii* pneumonia. HIV testing is positive and physician documentation supports HIV disease with pneumonia.

a. *Should the fever, weakness, and enlarged lymph nodes be coded?*

_____

_____

b. *What is the first listed diagnosis?*

_____

_____

c. *Code all the diagnoses for this case, listing the primary diagnosis first.*

_____

_____

INTERNET RESEARCH

1. Access the recommended HIV screening guidelines published by the Centers for Disease Control and Prevention at www.cdc.gov/mmwr/. Search the *Morbidity and Mortality Weekly Report* (MMWR) for "Revised Recommendations for HIV Testing." Identify ways in which these screening exams are completed in your state.
2. Research the different AIDS treatments at http://aidsinfo.nih.gov/, and classify the medications into specific categories. Discuss how AIDS-related disease affects treatment.
3. Visit www.cdc.gov/hiv/testing/clinical/index.html. Discuss the role of HIV rapid testing in the diagnosis and treatment of AIDS. What other tests are used to confirm the presence of the virus?
4. Visit www.medlineplus.gov, and research conditions, diseases, wellness, and prescription information by being directed to answers to your health questions.
5. Access the American College of Surgeons website www.facs.org/cancer/ncdb/publicaccess .html to identify the top malignant neoplasms in the country. Identify other unique facts and information located at this site regarding cancer programs.

MEDICAL CODING LAB Remember to use the coding activities at **Medicalcodinglab.com** for extra practice on what you have just learned and to test your knowledge.

CHAPTER 6

ICD-10-CM Chapters 6 Through 10: G00–J99

The ICD-10-CM Chapters 6 through 10 list the codes for disorders of the nervous system, sense organs, circulatory system, and respiratory system. Chapter 6 in *Conquer Medical Coding* explains the correct coding and sequencing of patients' diagnosed or suspected conditions involving these systems, such as cerebrovascular disease, as well as eye and ear disorders. In addition, the chapter explains the following topics:

- The general guidelines for coding pain and pain management, differentiating between visits to manage pain and visits to treat the underlying cause of pain
- The major points to consider in code selection and assignment for paralysis and for epilepsy
- The key points for coding hypertensive disease
- The assignment of initial and subsequent codes for acute myocardial infarction
- The steps in code assignment for various types of heart failure
- The coding and sequencing of chronic obstructive pulmonary disease (COPD) and asthma

CODE IT!

Assign all pertinent ICD-10-CM codes to the following diagnoses or conditions.

1. _____ Acute on chronic diastolic CHF
2. _____ Hypertensive heart disease with chronic renal failure stage IV
3. _____ Status asthmaticus with COPD
4. _____ Acute frontal and ethmoidal sinusitis caused by MRSA
5. _____ Bilateral hypertensive retinopathy
6. _____ Sensory hearing loss, bilateral
7. _____ Chronic recurrent mastoiditis in the right ear
8. _____ Episodic cluster headaches (intractable)
9. _____ Parkinson's disease with dementia
10. _____ Chronic abdominal aortic aneurysm

MULTIPLE CHOICE

Select the option that best completes the statement or answers the question.

1. Sandy visited the doctor to have her eyes checked. The doctor prescribed a change in glasses for her malignant myopia of both eyes. Irregular astigmatism and preglaucoma of both eyes were also noted on her medical record. How would this be coded?
   A. H44.23, H52.213, H40.003
   B. H44.20, H52.219, H40.003
   C. H44.23, H52.213, H40.009
   D. H53.13, H52.213, H40.009

2. Choose the correct coding assignment for a cerebral infarction caused by thrombosis of the right carotid artery.
   A. I63.032
   B. I63.031
   C. I63.011
   D. I63.019

3. A patient presents with aortic, tricuspid, and mitral valve insufficiency. How would this be coded?
   A. I08.8
   B. I34.8
   C. I08.9
   D. I08.3

4. What is the correct coding assignment for a patient who is admitted for control of postoperative neck pain?
   A. G89.18, M54.2
   B. G89.28, M54.2
   C. G89.18
   D. M54.2, G89.18

5. How would you code hypoxemic acute respiratory failure with COPD exacerbation?
   A. J44.1, J96.00
   B. J96.01, J44.1
   C. J96.01, J44.0
   D. J44.9

6. A patient has mitral valve stenosis with insufficiency, along with known biventricular heart failure. The patient also has chronic renal failure, stage II, and hypertension. How would you code this?
   A. I05.2, I50.82, I13.0, N18.2
   B. I05.2, I50.9, I12.0
   C. I05.0, I34.0, I12.9, I11.0, N18.2, I50.82
   D. I05.0, I08.0, I50.82, I13.0, N18.2

7. What is the correct code for metabolic toxic encephalopathy?
   A. G93.41
   B. G92
   C. G93.49
   D. G93.40

8. A patient's chest x-ray revealed a large, left-sided, spontaneous tension pneumothorax with a mediastinal shift. The patient indicates a 20 pack per year smoking history and continues to smoke cigarettes. What codes should be used?
   A. J93.9, F17.210
   B. J93.0, F17.200
   C. J93.0, F17.210
   D. J93.83, F17.210

9. Which medication could be used to treat atrial fibrillation (arrhythmia)?
   A. Beta blocker
   B. Diuretic
   C. Thrombolytic
   D. Streptokinase

10. The patient presents with shortness of breath and hemoptysis. Bronchoscopy is positive for obstruction in the left bronchial tree caused by pulmonary abscess. Culture is taken and is positive for *Klebsiella*. The attending physician states the diagnosis of acute right upper lobe *Klebsiella* pneumonia caused by abscess. What codes should be used?
    A. J85.1, J18.9, B96.1
    B. J85.1, J15.0, B96.1
    C. J85.2, B96.1
    D. J85.1, J15.0

SHORT ANSWER

Answer the following questions.

1. When reporting an acute myocardial infarction, what time period is considered when reporting a subsequent myocardial infarction?

   _____

   _____

2. The patient presents to the physician office with chest pain and has known coronary artery disease. The ECG is abnormal. Identify the medical condition reported first.

   _____

   _____

3. The patient has an upper GI bleed caused by gastritis. The patient's hemoglobin and hematocrit are low, and the patient receives a blood transfusion of packed cells. Does documentation support a causal relationship between the GI bleed and underlying cause?

   _____

   _____

4. What disease do we assume has a relationship to hypertension, even if the relationship is not stated?

   _____

   _____

5. According to the U.S. definitions, which categories of visual impairment denote blindness?

   _____

   _____

6. When is it appropriate to assign a code from G89 first, even if we know the underlying diagnosis?

   _____

   _____

7. What are some of the conditions included under the classification of COPD in ICD-10-CM?

_____

_____

8. What does it mean when there is an "exacerbation" of a condition?

_____

_____

9. Which type of anesthesia requires mechanical ventilation?

_____

_____

10. This right-handed patient suffered left-sided hemiplegia following a cerebral vascular accident. Considering the code for hemiplegia, is the dominant or nondominant side affected?

_____

_____

CASE STUDIES

1. Mitchell H.

   Office Note

   > **SUBJECTIVE:** Patient presents with general malaise, fever to 103, and cough occasionally productive of blood-tinged sputum for 1 day. He denies nausea or vomiting.
   > **OBJECTIVE:** Temperature, 102.7. He is in mild distress.
   > **HEENT:** Nares are patent. Pharynx is markedly erythematous without exudates or ulcerations.
   > **NECK:** Supple with shotty anterior cervical lymphadenopathy bilaterally.
   > **CHEST:** Examination reveals rare scattered rhonchi, which clear with cough.
   > **LAB:** Chest x-ray reveals no discrete infiltrates.
   > **ASSESSMENT:** Acute bronchitis with bronchospasm.
   > **PLAN:** Push fluids. Tylenol for fever. E.E.S. 400 mg QID x 10 days. Robitussin DM PRN cough. Follow up 3 days if symptoms do not improve.

   a. *What are the patient's signs and symptoms?*

   _____

   _____

   b. *Assign the ICD-10-CM codes.*

   _____

   _____

2. Myran P.

   Myran presents to Dr. Doe's office complaining that he has coughed up blood (hemoptysis) twice recently and has been short of breath. Myran is a heavy cigarette smoker, two packs per day × 40 years. Dr. Doe schedules Myran for a lung scan.

   Assign the ICD-10-CM code(s).

   _____

   _____

3. Emerson F.

Emerson is a white male who has a 1-month history of arm and chest discomfort. His symptoms occur with exertion and at rest. A stress echo done in August suggested posterior ischemia and an ejection fraction of 60%. Because of this, CCS class II unstable anginal symptoms, as well as risk factors of type 2 diabetes mellitus and mixed hyperlipidemia, he was referred for cardiac catheterization, which revealed a 75% occluded distal circumflex artery caused by arteriosclerosis.

a. *Which diagnostic tests confirmed the presence of coronary artery disease?*

_____

_____

b. *Assign the ICD-10-CM code(s).*

_____

_____

4. Carlos S.

Carlos is an alert, well-developed, well-nourished Hispanic male who used detergent at work and then accidentally rubbed his eyes, which became red and sore. Today, during the initial care, his right and left eyes are red, watery, and sealed shut with yellow discharge. Prescription was given for Gentamycin eyedrops. Diagnosis: Acute bilateral conjunctivitis, chemical induced.

a. *Which coding convention applies to reporting chemical conjunctivitis?*

_____

_____

b. *Assign the ICD-10-CM code(s).*

_____

_____

5. Selma A.

Selma, an ambulatory female, comes into the ED/OPD complaining of severe headache for 1 day, associated with numbness on the right side of the face and right arm. No neurovascular problems are associated with this, but the patient does have left eye photophobia. Diagnosis: Intractable tension headache.

Assign the ICD-10-CM code(s).

_____

_____

6. Juanita M.

Juanita states about 2 hours ago she got terrible chest and arm pain. Presently, the patient complains of severe substernal chest pain, right and left arm pain, and diaphoresis. EKG is positive for acute ST elevated inferior wall myocardial infarction.

Assign the ICD-10-CM code(s).

_____

_____

7. Elizabeth S.

The patient, an alert female, presents with bleeding from the right nares. She suffers from generalized arthritis, for which she takes Celebrex. She also has a long history of COPD, possibly related to tobacco dependence (she quit 5 years ago) but is now oxygen dependent.
FINAL DIAGNOSIS: Nosebleed, COPD, generalized osteoarthritis, and oxygen dependence.

a. *What is the medical term for nosebleed?*

_____

_____

b. *Assign the ICD-10-CM code(s).*

_____

_____

8. Lynda I.

Lynda presents to the outpatient pain clinic for epidural injection to manage her chronic low back pain caused by herniated lumbar discs at L3 through L5. The injections were given and the patient went home without incident.

a. *Which ICD-10-CM Official Guideline applies to the sequencing of the codes for this visit?*

_____

_____

b. *Assign the ICD-10-CM codes in the correct sequence.*

_____

_____

9. Jackson F.

> The patient is a black male with known hypertension and atrial fibrillation. The patient is on long-term Coumadin (anticoagulation) to treat the chronic arrhythmia. The patient now presents with facial droop, dysphasia, and flaccid left hemiplegia (the patient is left handed). MRI of the brain is positive for acute left posterior embolic cerebrovascular accident.
> **DIAGNOSES:** Acute CVA, hypertension, atrial fibrillation, long-term Coumadin use.

a. *List the neurological deficits from the cerebral embolism.*

_____

_____

b. *Assign the ICD-10-CM code(s).*

_____

_____

10. Marge O.

Marge is a female with a sick sinus syndrome and presents for pacemaker insertion. After admission, she developed chest pain with work-up supporting type 3 myocardial infarction.

a. *What is another name for sick sinus syndrome?*

_____

_____

b. *Assign the ICD-10-CM code(s).*

_____

_____

INTERNET RESEARCH

1. Access the tutorial on congestive heart failure at http://www.nhlbi.nih.gov/health/ health-topics. Select "Heart Failure" in the index and note the different causes of heart failure. Discuss how the cause of heart failure affects code assignment.

2. Visit www.webmd.com/heart-disease/electrocardiogram. Identify the different reasons an electrocardiogram (ECG) might be done—that is, identify the heart diseases that can be detected from an ECG. Follow the link to view a normal ECG tracing at "The spikes and dips in the line tracings are called waves." Click on the camera, which leads the reader to "EKG components and intervals."

3. Open the Joint Commission core measure set for acute myocardial infarction at www .jointcommission.org/core_measure_sets.aspx. Research the performance measures for acute myocardial infarction by clicking on "Acute Myocardial Infarction" from the list of Core Measure Sets.

MEDICAL CODING LAB Remember to use the coding activities at **Medicalcodinglab.com** for extra practice on what you have just learned and to test your knowledge.

CHAPTER 7

ICD-10-CM Chapters 11 Through 14: K00–N99

The ICD-10-CM Chapters 11 through 14 list the codes for diseases and disorders of the digestive, integumentary, musculoskeletal, and genitourinary systems. Chapter 7 in *Conquer Medical Coding* explains the correct coding and complex coding scenarios of patients' conditions involving these structures and systems such as gastrointestinal (GI) hemorrhage, skin ulcers, rheumatism, and kidney disease. In addition, the chapter explains the following topics:

- The general points relating to coding for digestive system disorders
- The four stages of pressure ulcers and why coding a pressure ulcer requires two ICD-10-CM codes
- The coding rules that apply for ischemic ulcers and for venous stasis ulcers
- The coding rule that governs coding of unstageable versus unspecified pressure ulcers
- The coding rules that apply for complications that have caused cellulitis and for gangrenous cellulitis
- The correct coding and sequencing for cellulitis
- The coding and sequencing of pathological fractures
- The coding of osteomyelitis and the unique rule for coding coexisting diabetes and osteomyelitis

CODE IT!

Assign all pertinent ICD-10-CM codes to the following diagnoses or conditions.

1. _____ Recurrent, *Clostridium difficile* enteritis

2. _____ Acute hepatic encephalopathy secondary to cirrhosis of the liver

3. _____ Acute and chronic diverticulitis of cecum with bacterial peritonitis

4. _____ Abdominal pain secondary to acute gallstone pancreatitis and acute cholelithiasis with acute cholecystitis

5. _____ Endometriosis of the uterus

6. _____ Intrinsic eczema

7. _____ Poison ivy

8. _____ Rheumatoid arthritis (seronegative)

9. _____ Urinary urgency and frequency

10. _____ Right hallux valgus and hammertoe

MULTIPLE CHOICE

Select the option that best provides the correct code, completes the statement, or answers the question.

1. What is the correct code for acute perforated gastric ulcer with hemorrhage? Patient is also diagnosed with blood loss anemia.
   A. K25.5, D62
   B. K25.0, D64.9
   C. K25.2, D50.0
   D. K25.5, D50.0

2. A 45-year-old inpatient was admitted with gastrointestinal bleeding. Colonoscopy revealed adenomatous polyp of the sigmoid, which was bleeding. Five days post-op, the patient developed a urinary tract infection caused by *E. coli*. What is the correct code?
   A. D12.5, K92.2, N39.0, B96.20
   B. D12.6, N39.0, A49.8
   C. D12.5, N39.0, B96.20
   D. D12.6, K92.2, N39.0, A49.8

3. Acute renal failure with renal medullary necrosis and hypertension is coded as:
   A. N17.9, I12.9
   B. N17.2, I10
   C. N17.0, I10
   D. N17.2, I12.9, N18.9

4. What is the correct coding for menometrorrhagia caused by uterine leiomyoma (subserosal)? The patient has chronic blood loss anemia, hypertension, and end-stage renal disease that requires hemodialysis.
   A. N92.1, D25.2, D50.0, I12.0, N18.6
   B. D25.2, D50.0, I12.0
   C. D25.2, N92.1, D50.0, I12.0, N18.6, Z99.2
   D. D25.2, N92.1, D50.0, I12.0, Z99.2

5. Epigastric pain caused by gastritis is coded as:
   A. R10.13, K29.70
   B. K29.70
   C. R10.9, K29.70
   D. K29.00

6. Type 1 diabetic peripheral vascular disease with right heel ulcer with muscle involvement without evidence of necrosis is coded as:
   A. E11.51, E11.622
   B. E10.51, E10.621
   C. E10.51, E10.622, L97.405
   D. E10.51, E10.621, L97.415

7. Initial care for pathological fracture of the lumbar vertebra secondary to idiopathic osteoporosis is coded as:
   A. M80.88xA
   B. M84.48xA
   C. M84.48xA, M81.0
   D. M80.88xA, M81.0

8. The patient has nonunion of right tibia pathological fracture with ankle pain. The patient also has cellulitis of the right ankle caused by MRSA. Report codes are:
   A. M84.461P, L03.115, A49.02
   B. M84.461K, A49.02
   C. M84.461P, L03.818, B95.62
   D. M84.461K, L03.115, B95.62

9. Stage II pressure ulcer of the right buttock is coded as:
   A. L89.302
   B. L89.310
   C. L89.312
   D. L89.300

10. The patient is an alcoholic who presents with left lower quadrant abdominal pain and abdominal ascites caused by acute alcoholic hepatitis. This is coded as:
   A. K70.11, R18.8, F10.21
   B. K70.11, F10.20
   C. K70.11, F10.20, R10.32
   D. K70.10, R18.8

SHORT ANSWER

Answer the following questions.

1. What are the clinical signs that a physician query is appropriate for this case? The patient has upper GI bleed caused by gastritis. The patient's hemoglobin and hematocrit are low, and the patient receives a blood transfusion of packed red blood cells. _____

   _____

   _____

2. Antifungal medication agents are used to treat what type of skin disease? _____

   _____

   _____

3. Documentation supports a decubitus ulcer, which involves full-thickness skin loss involving the subcutaneous tissue and a portion of the fascia. What stage is this decubitus ulcer?

   _____

   _____

4. What does the abbreviation RUE mean? _____

   _____

   _____

5. What does the abbreviation TAH mean? _____

   _____

   _____

6. Oxycontin, codeine, and methadone are all considered what type of analgesics? _____

_____

_____

7. If a patient has a glomerular filtration rate of 75, what stage of CKD does this patient have?

_____

_____

8. What column from the Table of Drugs and Chemicals would you use to report the code for
   allergic drug-induced dermatitis from correct usage of topical antibiotic cream? _____

_____

_____

9. What type of urinary medications act as bladder antispasmodics? _____

_____

_____

10. When reporting prostatic hypertrophy, the abbreviation LUTS refers to what symptoms? ____

_____

_____

CASE STUDIES

1. Richard G.

> **SUBJECTIVE:** Richard is a 15-year-old male with increasing acne over the last 1 to 2 years. He has
> been using soap and Oxy-10 without improvement.
> **OBJECTIVE:** On the face, neck, and upper back, there is mild to moderate acne. Lesions consist of
> macules, papules, mild oily comedos, and an occasional nodule, but no cysts or boils. There is
> some scarring.
> **ASSESSMENT:** Acne vulgaris, mild to moderate with acne keloid.
> **PLAN:** Oxy-10. Retin A 0.25 mg cream applied sparingly to facial lesions. E.E.S. 400 mg TID x 3
> months. Recheck in 3 months.

Assign the diagnosis code or codes for this visit. _____

2. Sarah T.

> **SUBJECTIVE:** Patient presents with mild urinary frequency and some lower periumbilical abdomi-
> nal pain. She has no vaginal symptoms.
> **OBJECTIVE:** There is mild suprapubic tenderness; otherwise, examination is unremarkable.
> **LAB:** Urinalysis is negative, but quite dilute from increased fluid intake.
> **ASSESSMENT:** Urethritis.
> **PLAN:** Placed on 3-day course of Macrodantin. Recheck if not improving.

a. *What are the patient's signs and symptoms?* _____

_____

_____

b. *Assign the ICD-10-CM code(s).* _____

3. Bridget B.

Bridget visited Dr. Doe complaining of frequency and burning on urination. She also has lower abdominal pain. Urinalysis reveals many bacteria. Dr. Doe prescribes antibiotics and records a diagnosis of acute cystitis on her medical record. He also evaluated her hypertensive heart disease and noted no signs of failure, so no changes were made in her medication.

Assign the ICD-10-CM code(s). _____

4. Norm K.

Norm was admitted with localized primary osteoarthritis of the left knee. Norm also has gouty arthritis which requires medication and type 2 insulin-dependent diabetes mellitus.

Assign the ICD-10-CM code(s). _____

5. Rosa

Rosa is a female admitted with weakness, chest pain, and nausea with vomiting. Upper endoscopy with biopsy revealed an acute bleeding duodenal ulcer as the cause of all her symptoms. Her hemoglobin and hematocrit were low and the physician documents acute blood loss anemia. Rosa also has right hemiplegia and expressive aphasia caused by an old cerebral infarction that increased nursing care.

a. *Which condition in this case is considered a sequelae?* _____

_____

b. *Assign the ICD-10-CM code(s).* _____

6. Melvin R.

Melvin was scheduled for a laparoscopic cholecystectomy for cholecystitis. However, upon starting the laparoscopy, an open cholecystectomy and common bile duct exploration had to be performed because of acute cholecystitis with choledocholithiasis.

a. *To what cross reference is the coder directed when looking up the main term* choledocholithiasis?

_____

b. *Assign the ICD-10-CM code(s).* _____

7. Jason C.

> A patient with known Crohn's disease of the large intestine presented with small bowel obstruction and bloody stool. Upon admission, the patient had digestive decompression via NG tube and required total parenteral nutrition for 3 days. CT scan of the abdomen was positive for Crohn's disease localized in the jejunum and cecum.
> **DIAGNOSIS:** Small bowel obstruction and rectal bleeding caused by Crohn's disease.

a. *Is the cecum located in the large or small intestine?* _____

b. *Assign the ICD-10-CM code(s).* _____

8. Zelda G.

> The patient presents with menorrhagia and pelvic pain. As a result, she has developed anemia. The patient underwent scheduled total abdominal hysterectomy (TAH) and pathology results noted multiple subserous leiomyomas and adenoma of the left ovary. The patient also received two units of packed cells for anemia.
>
> **DIAGNOSIS:** Uterine fibroid, ovarian adenoma, and chronic anemia. Note: Physician was queried to determine if anemia was caused by chronic blood loss and he confirmed that anemia was specifically chronic blood loss anemia caused by fibroids.

Assign the ICD-10-CM code(s). _____

9. Shelly W.

> **POSTOPERATIVE DIAGNOSIS:** Symptomatic large endometrial polyp.
> **OPERATION:** Hysteroscopy, dilation and curettage.
> Examination under anesthesia. The cervix was pulled forward and was found to be patulous and easily admitted a 3-mm 30-degree hysteroscope attached to 1.5% Glycine. On hysteroscopy, a very large endometrial polyp was encountered. The polyp was removed with curettage and the ureteral stone forceps. Curettage revealed a moderate amount of tissue, as well. Endometrial curetting was then performed with a small, sharp serrated curet and a large sharp curet. Moderate tissue was obtained.

Assign the ICD-10-CM code(s). _____

10. Fraser T.

> **DIAGNOSIS:** Bladder cancer.
> **PROCEDURE:** Cystoscopy with bladder biopsies and fulguration.
> On rectal examination, the prostate gland is 20 grams, smooth and firm, and there are no rectal masses. A #21 French panendoscope was then introduced into the bladder. At cystoscopy, the urethra appears normal. The prostatic fossa has some moderate obstruction. The bladder itself contains no foreign bodies or stones. At the right dome of the bladder, and along the right bladder wall, three separate areas were identified with irregular mucosa, each measuring 0.5 cm. Bladder biopsies were taken and these areas were fulgurated.
> **PATHOLOGY REPORT:** Confirmed the diagnosis of overlapping transitional cell carcinoma of the bladder (dome and wall).

Assign the ICD-10-CM code(s). _____

INTERNET RESEARCH

1. Osteoarthritis can lead to pathological fractures. Go to www.mayoclinic.org/diseases-conditions, and research the prevention and control of osteoarthritis.

2. Access www.merck.com/mmhe/sec18.html to see a glossary of skin disorders and how they are categorized (cancers, infections, etc.). Research the signs, symptoms, prevention, and treatment of five skin disorders. You can also try to code them.

MEDICAL CODING LAB Remember to use the coding activities at **Medicalcodinglab.com** for extra practice on what you have just learned and to test your knowledge.

CHAPTER 8

ICD-10-CM Chapters 15 Through 17: O00–Q99

The ICD-10-CM Chapters 15 through 17 list the codes for conditions and disorders associated with pregnancy; childbirth; the perinatal period; and congenital malformations, deformations, and chromosomal abnormalities. Chapter 8 in *Conquer Medical Coding* explains the correct coding and complex coding scenarios of patients' conditions involving these events, conditions, and complications, such as HIV infection in pregnancy and diabetes related to pregnancy. Correct code assignment and sequencing of complications require careful review of the guidelines because these conditions have sequencing priority over codes from the other ICD-10-CM chapters. Chapter 8 also covers the following topics:

- The correct use of the final character, which classifies the trimester
- The seventh character for fetus identification in certain categories
- The differences among preexisting conditions versus conditions caused by the pregnancy
- The purpose and correct assignment of outcome of delivery codes, including a normal delivery or an abortive outcome
- The implications for future health-care needs when coding perinatal conditions
- The coding of community-acquired conditions in the perinatal period
- The coding guidelines for perinatal conditions resulting from maternal factors (category P00–P04)

CODE IT!

Assign all pertinent ICD-10-CM codes to the following diagnoses or conditions.

1. _____ Routine postpartum visit

2. _____ Newborn jaundice caused by ABO incompatibility

3. _____ Fourteen-day-old infant evaluated for suspected sepsis caused by fever; sepsis ruled out

4. _____ Single newborn delivered via cesarean section; the newborn tests positive for heroin

5. _____ Newborn admitted at age 10 days, because of coarctation of the pulmonary artery

6. _____ Type 2 insulin-dependent diabetic mother, now admitted for diabetic ketoacidosis at 22 weeks' gestation

7. _____ Pregnancy at 37 weeks' gestation with arrested active phase and fetal bradycardia that required cesarean section; a single live-born was delivered

8. _____ A 25-year-old female delivered full-term dichorionic, diamniotic live-born twins at 38 weeks via low forceps following failed vacuum extraction

9. _____ Eighteen-day-old infant admitted because of community-acquired pneumonia and esophageal reflux

10. _____ The outcome of delivery code for Sheila who was discharged following delivery of twins, one live-born, one stillborn

MULTIPLE CHOICE

Select the option that best provides the correct code, completes the statement, or answers the question.

1. Cervical incompetence at 24 weeks' gestation is coded as:
   A. O34.30
   B. N88.3
   C. O34.32, Z3A.24
   D. O34.32

2. Hypoglycemia in an infant of a diabetic mother is coded as:
   A. P70.1
   B. P70.0, Z38.00
   C. P70.1, Z38.00
   D. P70.0

3. Postpartum breast abscess is coded as:
   A. O91.13, N61
   B. O91.12, N61
   C. O91.13
   D. O91.12

4. Induction of labor because of intrauterine fetal demise at 25 weeks, with stillborn birth, is coded as:
   A. O02.1, Z3A.25
   B. O36.4xx0, Z37.1, Z3A.25
   C. O36.4xx0, Z37.7, Z3A.25
   D. O02.1, Z37.1, Z3A.25

5. Newborn failure to thrive, RSV bronchiolitis (infection) at 20 days of life, is coded as:
   A. P92.6, P39.8, J21.0
   B. P92.6, J21.0
   C. P92.6, P39.9, J21.0
   D. P62.51, P39.9

6. The patient presents with pregnancy, complicated by acquired hemolytic anemia and depression. A full-term baby girl was delivered at 38 weeks. Report codes as:
   A. O99.02, D59.9, O99.343, Z37.0, Z3A.38
   B. O99.02, D59.9, O99.344, F32.9, Z37.0, Z3A.38
   C. O99.02, D58.9, O99.344, Z37.0, Z3A.38
   D. O99.02, O99.343, Z37.0, Z3A.38

7. A 24-year-old female has a vaginal delivery of her monochorionic, diamniotic twins prematurely at 32 weeks with precipitate labor. The first fetus is treated for fetal growth retardation. Report codes as:
   A. O30.033, O60.14x0, O36.5910, O62.3, Z37.2, Z3A.32
   B. O30.033, O60.14x1, O36.5911, O62.3, Z37.2, Z3A.32
   C. O30.033, O60.14x1, O60.14x2, P28, Z37.2, Z3A.32
   D. O30.033, O60.14x1, O60.14x2, O36.5911, O62.3, Z37.2, Z3A.32

8. Newborn triplets are delivered vaginally at 32 weeks (premature). Baby number 2 weighs 1,800 grams with a heart murmur from Tetralogy of Fallot. Report codes as:
   A. Z38.61, P07.35, P07.17, Q21.3
   B. Z38.61, P07.35, Q21.3
   C. P07.35, P07.17, Q21.3
   D. Z38.61, P07.35, P07.17, R01.1

9. A 40-year-old woman presents for her prenatal visit in her 21st week. This is a high-risk pregnancy because of her elderly primigravida status and gestational hypertension which developed at 12 weeks. Report codes as:
   A. O09.512, O13.1
   B. O09.512, O13.2, Z3A.21
   C. O09.512, O13.1, Z3A.21
   D. O09.512, O16.2, I10, Z3A.21

10. Positive pregnancy test is coded as:
    A. Z32.00
    B. Z32.01
    C. Z32.02
    D. Z32.01, O80

SHORT ANSWER

Answer the following questions.

1. What is the name of the drug or chemical used to treat apnea of prematurity? _____
   _____
   _____

2. What drug is used to prevent respiratory distress syndrome (RDS) in newborns?_____
   _____
   _____

3. What types of drugs are used to suppress contractions associated with premature labor?
   _____
   _____

4. What type of abortion can also be called a miscarriage? _____
   _____
   _____

5. What is the normal duration of the postpartum period? _____

_____

_____

6. If a patient is seen at 32 weeks for an obstetrical problem, which trimester is the patient in?

_____

_____

7. If the obstetrical problem is breech presentation of a single fetus, what is the appropriate seventh character for the code O32.1xx? _____

_____

8. Can the code O80 and Z37.2 be reported together? If not, please explain. _____

_____

_____

9. When reporting an obstetrical laceration during delivery, what present on admission indicator would be assigned? _____

_____

_____

CASE STUDIES

For Questions 1 through 5, report the codes for both the mother and baby where appropriate.

1. Alice B.

   Alice, a 38-year-old elderly primigravida, presented with premature labor at 35 weeks' gestation with placenta previa. A single live-born female was delivered vaginally over an intact perineum. The baby weighed 1,900 grams.

   a. *Mother's record:* _____

   b. *Baby's record:* _____

2. Rupa S.

   Rupa, a 22-year-old female, presented with premature monochorionic, diamniotic twin pregnancy at 36 weeks' gestation. The babies were delivered via low transverse cesarean section because of fetal bradycardia from twin A. Twin A weighed 2,100 grams, and twin B weighed 2,000 grams.

   a. *Mother's record:* _____

   b. *Baby A's record:* _____

   c. *Baby B's record:* _____

3. Mary E.

   Mary presented in preterm labor at 33 weeks. Tocolytics were provided, which stopped the contractions. Mary has a history of preterm labor and went home on bed rest.

   Assign the ICD-10-CM code(s). _____

4. Jenny L.

Jenny had a postdate pregnancy at 41 weeks and was admitted for surgical induction of labor. Jenny has a history of previous cesarean delivery caused by preterm labor in the third trimester. Her child, a single large-for-gestational-age boy, required delivery by cesarean section.

   a. *Mother's record:* _____

   b. *Baby's record:* _____

5. Xaiodan B.

Xaiodan, a premature baby born at 32 weeks, presents for his first newborn care office visit at 6 days old. The birth weight was 1,600 grams.

Assign the ICD-10-CM code(s). _____

6. Maureen O.

Maureen was discharged 2 days ago following dilation and curettage (D&C) for a spontaneous abortion. Today, she is admitted with pelvic peritonitis. Culture is positive for *Staphylococcus aureus*.

Assign the ICD-10-CM code(s). _____

7. Mirimar L.

> The patient, a 26-year-old female, presented because of pregnancy-induced hypertension with severe preeclampsia at 34 weeks' gestation. Medical induction of labor was begun and the patient required low transverse cesarean section because of fetal bradycardia. Two days after cesarean delivery, it was noted that the patient developed postoperative acute blood loss anemia. The patient delivered a 34-week-old single live-born male.
> **DIAGNOSIS:** Pregnancy-induced hypertension with severe preeclampsia, premature delivery, and cesarean section because of fetal bradycardia and post-op anemia.

   a. *Mother's record:* _____

   b. *Baby's record:* _____

8. Marnesha W.

Marnesha, a 24-year-old female, presents at 39 weeks with normal spontaneous vaginal delivery of a single live-born infant. There were no pregnancy complications. The patient requested tubal ligation for sterilization.

   a. *Mother's record:* _____

   b. *Baby's record:* _____

9. Amardeep L.

Amardeep's triplet pregnancy at 37 weeks was complicated by preexisting type 1 diabetes and GBS-positive status. All three babies were delivered vaginally without complications.

   a. *Mother's record:* _____

   b. *Baby A, B, and C record:* _____

10. Amy S.

Live-born twin A (mate live-born) was delivered via cesarean section at 39 weeks. Hospitalization was complicated by *E. coli* sepsis, apnea, and baby born "light-for-dates." Birth weight was 2,211 grams.

Assign ICD-10-CM code(s) for baby A. _____

INTERNET RESEARCH

1. Go to www.doh.wa.gov/Portals/1/Documents/Pubs/birthdefects.pdf, which contains the birth defects list of notifiable conditions for the Washington State Birth Defects Surveillance System. Take note of the conditions that require reporting. Locate the list of reportable birth defects for your state.
2. Review the reVITALize obstetric data definitions from the American Congress of Obstetricians and Gynecologists at http://www.acog.org and search for Obstetric Data Definitions. Choose one category of definitions to research (e.g., gestational age and term). What are the benefits of creating these data definitions?

MEDICAL CODING LAB Remember to use the coding activities at **Medicalcodinglab.com** for extra practice on what you have just learned and to test your knowledge.

CHAPTER 9

ICD-10-CM Chapters 18 Through 21: R00–Z99

The ICD-10-CM Chapters 18 through 22 list the codes involving symptoms, signs, and abnormal clinical and laboratory findings not elsewhere classified; injuries, poisoning, and certain other consequences of external causes; external causes of morbidity; and factors influencing health status and contact with health service. Chapter 9 in *Conquer Medical Coding* explains the correct coding and complex coding scenarios for these cases. For example, each injury, whether it is a single injury or one of multiple injuries, is assigned a separate code. Burns require two codes: a code for the burn's body site and severity, and a second code for its extent. To code a condition as a complication, documentation must state a causal relationship between the condition and the medical care or procedure. In general, reporting of sign and symptom codes requires knowledge of the disease process. The chapter also explains the following topics:

- The difference between the coding rules for integral and nonintegral signs and symptoms
- The difference in the way signs and symptoms are reported in the inpatient setting versus the outpatient setting
- The general guidelines for coding injuries
- The coding of adverse effects
- The definition of poisoning as used in ICD-10-CM coding, and the steps for coding this condition
- The definition of toxic effects as used in ICD-10-CM, and description of the steps for coding these events
- The general guidelines for coding complications of care
- The assignment of external cause codes for inpatient (facility) coding

CODE IT!

Assign all pertinent ICD-10-CM codes to the following diagnoses or conditions.

1. _____ Screening colonoscopy positive for sigmoid diverticulitis

2. _____ Admission for radiation therapy to treat bone metastasis; patient has history of prostate cancer

3. _____ Encounter for influenza vaccine

4. _____ Acute renal failure caused by kidney transplant rejection

5. _____ Second- and third-degree burns of the left upper arm (less than 10%) from leaning on hot car radiator at work in car factory

6. _____ Encounter for COPD exacerbation, ventilator dependent

7. _____ Upper gastrointestinal bleeding caused by adverse effect of Coumadin, initial care

8. _____ Observation for suspected maternal oligohydramnios, in third trimester, condition not found

9. _____ Periprosthetic left prosthetic hip fracture (initial episode)

10. _____ Postoperative bleeding from tonsillectomy site

MULTIPLE CHOICE

Select the option that best completes the statement or answers the question.

1. What is the correct coding assignment for a patient with a grand mal seizure disorder caused by the late effect (sequelae) of digoxin overdose in a previous suicide attempt?
   A. G40.409, T46.0X2S
   B. G40.419, T46.0X2S
   C. G40.409
   D. G40.909, T46.0X2A

2. How would you code a single-born infant, born via spontaneous vaginal delivery in the hospital, observed for suspected sepsis, which is ruled out?
   A. Z38.01, P36.9
   B. Z38.00, Z05.01
   C. P00.2
   D. Z38.00, P36.9

3. What is the correct coding assignment for a pre-op cardiovascular examination for a patient scheduled for inguinal hernia repair and who has hypertension and hypercholesterolemia?
   A. Z01.818, K40.90, I10, E78.0
   B. Z01.810, K40.90
   C. K40.90, I10, E78.0
   D. Z01.810, K40.90, I10, E78.0

4. What codes would you assign for a patient with third-degree burns of the lower left leg (5%) and first- and second-degree burns of the left forearm (3%) (do not report external cause codes)?
   A. T24.332A, T22.212A, T31.0
   B. T24.302A, T22.221A, T31.10
   C. T24.339A, T22.219A, T31.0
   D. T24.332A, T24.333A, T31.10

5. The patient presents to the emergency room with left shoulder pain. He fell off a skateboard and landed on his left side while he was at the park. X-ray showed Salter Type II fracture of the physeal end of the upper humerus.
   A. S49.012A, V00.132A, Y92.830
   B. S49.022A, V00.131A, Y92.830, Y93.51
   C. S49.122A, V00.131A, Y92.830, Y93.51
   D. S42.202A, V00.132A, Y92.830, Y93.51

6. What is the correct way to code an initial encounter for a patient with mechanical displacement of an autonomic implantable cardiodefibrillation (AICD) electrode?
   A. T82.129A
   B. T82.120A, Y83.1
   C. T82.129A, Y83.1
   D. T82.121A, Y83.1

7. The patient presented to the hospital with hemoptysis, gastrointestinal bleeding, and hematuria. Further workup was positive for an abnormal coagulation profile. Diagnosis: Bleeding caused by the adverse effects of Coumadin, abnormal coagulation profile. What is the correct way to code this situation?
   A. T45.515A, R04.2, K92.2, R31.9
   B. R04.2, K92.2, R31.9, D68.9, T45.516A
   C. R04.2, K92.2, R31.9, R79.1, T45.515A
   D. T45.515A, R79.1

8. The patient presents with a new seizure. He also has right flaccid hemiplegia (patient is right handed) and a previous Type II occipital condyle skull fracture after falling off a ladder at home 3 years ago. What is the correct way to code this situation?
   A. R56.9, G81.03, Z87.81, W11.xxxS
   B. R56.9, G81.01, W11.xxxS
   C. R56.9, I69.851, Z87.81
   D. R56.9, G81.01, S02.11ES, W11.xxxS, Y92.0009

9. A lone bicyclist sustained a severe laceration of the scalp after being struck by a car on a state road. Large amounts of gravel were removed from the wound. What is the correct way to code this situation?
   A. S01.02XA, V13.4XXA, Y92.412
   B. S01.01XA, V13.9XXA
   C. S01.02XA, V13.2XXA
   D. S01.01XA, V13.4XXA, Y92.412

10. The patient has an annual gynecological examination with an abnormal finding of a right breast mass. What is the correct way to code this situation?
    A. Z01.419, N63.10
    B. Z01.411, N63.10
    C. Z04.411, N60.01
    D. Z00.01, N63.14

SHORT ANSWER

Answer the following questions.

1. When reporting traumatic fractures in ICD-10-CM, is a fracture assumed to be displaced or nondisplaced? _____

2. Does the following diagnostic statement support the presence of a complication? If not, explain. "Urinary tract infection, patient has indwelling urinary catheter."_____

   _____

   _____

3. According to the rule of nines used to classify burns, what percentage of the adult body is burned if the entire left leg is involved? _____

4. A patient treated with acetylcysteine would be experiencing an overdose of which type of drug? _____

   _____

5. According to coding guidelines, which diagnosis would be reported first if a patient presents with an acute exacerbation of asthma because of an underdose of Flovent? _____

   _____

6. Identify this situation as either a poisoning or adverse effect: The patient presents with hematemesis following ingestion of red wine and Naprosyn. _____

_____

7. What are the three components of the Glasgow coma score? _____

_____

_____

8. What is the seventh character for a patient who presents to rehabilitation following treatment for a right hip fracture? _____

_____

9. Is the sign of right lower quadrant abdominal pain integral to appendicitis? _____

_____

10. External cause of injury codes are used to classify the mechanism of injury, place of injury, patient status, and: _____

CASE STUDIES

1. Tracylin I.

   Tracylin, a 30-year-old female, was admitted for prophylactic breast removal because of a family history of breast cancer. After surgery, Tracylin developed a postoperative wound infection caused by *Staphylococcus aureus*.

   a. *What is the external cause of injury code for the complication?* _____

   b. *Assign the ICD-10-CM code(s).* _____

2. Bubba S.

   Bubba, a 22-year-old male, lost control of his ATV while he was driving and hit a tree. He was admitted with a frontal skull fracture, cerebral contusion, and loss of consciousness for 48 hours. Bubba regained normal consciousness later. He also sustained a left lung contusion and minor liver laceration.

   a. *What main term is used to report the ATC accident?* _____

   b. *Assign the ICD-10-CM code(s).* _____

3. John D.

   John was found unconscious in his apartment and was brought to the emergency department (ED). Medical investigation revealed a positive blood test for cocaine, alcohol, and barbiturates. The patient was admitted and remained comatose until passing away on the fifth hospital day.

   a. *What is the external cause of injury code for place of occurrence?* _____

   b. *Would this case be considered an adverse reaction or poisoning?* _____

   _____

   c. *Assign the ICD-10-CM code(s).* _____

4. Krystin P.

Krystin was admitted for small bowel obstruction caused by anastomosis complication. After surgery for revision of anastomosis, she developed postoperative seroma of the skin near the incision site.

a. *Assign the ICD-10-CM principal diagnosis code.* _____

b. *Assign the additional ICD-10-CM codes.* _____

5. Antoinette M.

Antoinette was admitted for dehydration and neutropenia caused by chemotherapy (antineoplastic). The patient has known carcinoma of the sigmoid colon with liver metastasis. The patient required blood transfusion and IV fluids. During the blood transfusion, the patient developed the transfusion reaction of acute congestive heart failure.

a. *Is the complication of the chemotherapy a poisoning or adverse reaction?* _____

_____

b. *What is the primary site of the malignancy?*_____

_____

c. *Assign* the ICD-10-CM *codes sequencing the principal diagnosis first.*

_____

6. Alex D.

Alex was admitted after suffering from a depressed fracture of the occiput. Lumbar puncture revealed that subdural hemorrhage had resulted. The depressed fragments were surgically elevated.

a. *What additional documentation should be provided to completely code this case?* _____

_____

b. *Assign the ICD-10-CM code(s).* _____

7. Aaron R.

Aaron came to the ED with a bite wound of his right index finger involving the nail, bite wound of the dorsal aspect of the right hand, and a dislocated metacarpophalangeal joint of his right ring finger. He was bit by the neighbor's dog while in the back yard of their single family house.

a. *What conditions are excluded from the ICD-10-CM code for hand bite?* _____

_____

_____

b. *Assign the ICD-10-CM code(s).* _____

8. Gregory M.

Gregory reported to the ED complaining of severe headache, nausea, and photophobia following a severe hit on the head with a hockey puck while playing ice hockey. There was an LOC for 2 minutes. Neurological examination was noted to be as follows: Eyes open to sound, with a confused verbal response, and motor response in which he follows commands. After examination, the doctor concluded that Gregory has a brain concussion.

a. *Assign the ICD-10-CM codes for the Glasgow coma score.* _____

b. *Assign the ICD-10-CM external cause codes.* _____

c. *What additional code would be assigned, if documented, when reporting the concussion?*

_____

_____

d. *Assign the ICD-10-CM code for the concussion.* _____

9. Ramon V.

Ramon was seen for routine outpatient renal dialysis. He has end-stage CKD that requires dialysis on Mondays, Wednesdays, and Fridays. In the dialysis unit, it was noted his left forearm AV fistula was infected with a surrounding area of cellulitis. He is awaiting a kidney transplant.

a. *What is the meaning of the abbreviation CKD?* _____

_____

b. *Does documentation support a complication of the AV fistula?*

_____

c. *Assign the ICD-10-CM code(s).* _____

10. Mimi L.

Mimi presented to the physician office complaining of shortness of breath, wheezing, and itching. She also has a previous laceration of the right forearm that was healing from treatment with penicillin. The laceration was from the time she cut herself with a kitchen knife. She had stopped taking her COPD medication because of financial hardship. After evaluation, the following diagnoses were established: acute COPD exacerbation caused by underdosing of bronchodilators, allergic reaction to penicillin, healing laceration of the right forearm.

a. *What are the patient's symptoms?* _____

_____

_____

b. *Are any of the symptoms related to a medication?* _____

c. *What is the seventh character assigned for the laceration?* _____

d. *Assign the ICD-10-CM code(s) in the correct seque*nce. _____

INTERNET RESOURCES

1. Access the website http://www.ahrq.gov/topics/index.html, which provides a variety of articles on health-care quality. Research articles regarding complications following surgery. Do you think articles like the one you chose utilized ICD-10-CM codes to determine the rate of postoperative complications? Why or why not?
2. Access the website www.cdc.gov/safechild/playground/index.html, which reports playground injuries and deaths. What impact, if any, does reporting of external cause codes have on these national statistics? Find another report at the Centers for Disease Control and Prevention website that describes how injuries occur and the related number of deaths (i.e., motor vehicle accidents).

MEDICAL CODING LAB Remember to use the coding activities at **Medicalcodinglab.com** for extra practice on what you have just learned and to test your knowledge.

ICD-10-CM Outpatient Coding Guidelines

Chapter 10 in *Conquer Medical Coding* explains outpatient coding and reporting guidelines, determining first-listed diagnosis, and coding secondary diagnoses and external causes in outpatient settings. An outpatient is a patient who is not admitted to an acute care facility, short-term hospital, or any other inpatient setting; outpatients receive care from a facility and typically return home the same day. In the outpatient setting, the first-listed diagnosis is the reason for the visit, whether it is for a medical condition, screening, well visit, routine testing, immunization, or other reason. These guidelines are different from inpatient guidelines in many cases. For example, inconclusive conditions—those that are documented as possible, probable, or suspected—are not assigned codes in outpatient settings. A code is assigned for the condition, sign, or symptom that is known at the time of the visit. It is important that you understand thoroughly the intricacies of these codes because the majority of health-care patients' visits are to outpatient settings. Chapter 10 also explains the following topics:

- The diagnosis code sequencing rules for a variety of outpatient encounters, such as outpatient procedures or ambulatory surgeries, observation stays, and encounters for circumstances other than disease or injury
- The coding for uncertain conditions in the outpatient and inpatient settings
- The coding for chronic diseases in the outpatient setting
- The application of ICD-10-CM coding guidelines to outpatient visits when patients receive only diagnostic services, therapeutic services, or preoperative examinations.
- The application of outpatient coding guidelines for emergency department visits
- The coding and sequencing guidelines for routine outpatient prenatal visits
- The guidelines regarding reporting of additional diagnoses and E codes in the outpatient setting

CODE IT!

Assign all pertinent ICD-10-CM codes to the following diagnoses or conditions.

1. _____ Left lower quadrant abdominal pain, possible acute appendicitis

2. _____ Second-degree sunburn

3. _____ Chronic venous stasis left heel ulcer with varicose veins and muscle necrosis

4. _____ Patient who presents for outpatient colonoscopy caused by melena and family history of colon cancer

5. _____ Headache caused by acute bilateral frontal sinusitis

6. _____ Speech therapy visit for dysphasia from previous embolic CVA

7. _____ Twelve-year-old who presents to the physician office for physical examination for camp

8. _____ Observation for COPD exacerbation; patient has type 1 diabetes

9. _____ Patient sent for left ankle x-ray; patient has pain and diagnosis is possible fracture

10. _____ Ambulatory surgery for chronic cholecystitis; the patient requires observation for postoperative pain

MULTIPLE CHOICE

Select the option that best provides the correct code, completes the statement, or answers the question.

1. The patient presents to the obstetrician office because of hyperemesis gravidarum. The patient is 16 weeks' pregnant. What is the correct way to code this situation?
   A. Z34.02, O21.1, Z3A.16
   B. Z34.82, O21.0, Z3A.16
   C. O21.0, Z3A.16
   D. O21.0

2. The patient presents for post-op aftercare from traumatic bucket handle tear of the left medial and lateral meniscus. What is the correct way to code this situation?
   A. S83.252D, S83.212D
   B. Z47.89, S83.252D, S83.212D
   C. S83.252S, S83.212S
   D. Z47.89, S83.252A, S83.212A

3. Initial care was provided for a lacerated extensor tendon of the left ring finger caused by an automatic nail gun injury while building a new house at a construction site. What is the correct way to code this situation?
   A. S56.422A, W45.0XXA, Y92.69
   B. S66.321A, W29.4XXA, Y92.61
   C. S66.321A, W29.4XXA, Y92.69
   D. S66.422A, W29.4XXA, Y92.61

4. The patient has a 6-month check-up with vaccination for hepatitis B. The vaccine for chicken pox was not given because of the parent's wishes. What is the correct way to code this situation?
   A. Z00.121, Z23, Z28.82
   B. Z00.129, Z23
   C. Z00.121, Z28.82
   D. Z00.121, Z28.82

5. The patient presents with left foot pain probably caused by plantar fasciitis. What is the correct way to code this situation?
   A. M72.2
   B. M79.675, M72.2
   C. M79.672, M72.2
   D. M79.672

6. The patient has a severe rash caused by poison ivy. What is the correct way to code this situation?
   A. L23.7, R21
   B. R21
   C. L23.7
   D. L23.7, J30.1

7. A 25-year-old patient presents to the gynecologist because of an irregular menstrual cycle and inability to conceive. What is the correct way to code this situation?
   A. N92.1, N88.3
   B. N92.6, N97.9
   C. N92.6, N88.3
   D. N92.5, N97.9

8. A patient presented for chemotherapy to treat non-Hodgkin's lymphoma of the abdominal cavity and intrathoracic lymph nodes. Chemotherapy was cancelled because of findings of neutropenia. What is the correct way to code this situation?
   A. Z51.11, C85.98, D70.9, Z53.09
   B. Z51.11, C85.92, C85.93, D70.9
   C. C85.98, D70.4, Z53.09
   D. C85.92, C85.93, D70.4, D53.09

9. The patient has left lower quadrant abdominal pain and diarrhea caused by celiac disease with associated gluten ataxia. What is the correct way to code this situation?
   A. K90.0, R10.32, R197
   B. K90.0, R10.30, R19.7
   C. K90.0, R10.30, R19.7, G32.81
   D. K90.0, G32.81

10. A patient presents with chest pain, which is caused by anxiety. What is the correct way to code this situation?
    A. F41.9, R07.9
    B. F41.9, R07.89
    C. R07.9, F41.1
    D. F41.1, R07.89

SHORT ANSWER

Answer the following questions.

1. Would an observation patient be considered an inpatient or an outpatient? _____

   _____

2. Which diagnosis would be sequenced first for an ambulatory surgery patient who required an inguinal hernia repair and then observation services for postoperative nausea and vomiting? _____

   _____

3. Are external cause of injury codes reported for facility ED visits? _____

   _____

4. The code reported first in the outpatient setting is termed: _____

   _____

5. The code reported first in the inpatient setting is termed: _____

_____

6. May codes from Z00–Z99 be sequenced first in the outpatient setting? _____

_____

7. An ED visit contains the diagnostic impression of weakness, fever, and flank pain; rule out urinary tract infection. Which diagnoses would be reported? _____

_____

8. If a patient presents for a screening colonoscopy and a polyp is found, which diagnosis would be listed first? _____

_____

9. If a 36-year-old primigravida patient presents for a routine prenatal visit at 22 weeks, but has a high-risk pregnancy, which code would be reported first, code Z34.02 or O09.512? _____

_____

10. Which specific section of the *ICD-10-CM Official Guidelines for Coding and Reporting* instructs the coder to not report conditions that are no longer present or treated? _____

_____

CASE SCENARIOS

1. Henry H.

   Henry arrived for his physician office visit for hypertension, chronic atrial fibrillation, and COPD. The flu vaccine was also given.

   Assign the ICD-10-CM code(s). _____

2. Marlo D.

   Marlo presented for preoperative clearance for his upcoming knee surgery. He has a chronic tear of the right medial meniscus. After the physician noted that Marlo's type 1 diabetic neuropathy was controlled, he was cleared for surgery.

   a. *What is the first listed diagnosis code?* _____

   b. *Assign any additional ICD-10-CM codes.* _____

3. Luella O.

   Luella presented to the ED with acute alcohol intoxication (blood alcohol level is 102 mg/100 mL). Further evaluation was positive for hyponatremia and the patient was placed in observation for sodium supplementation with hydration.

   Assign the ICD-10-CM code(s). _____

4. Susan W.

   Susan presented to the Urgent Care Center with complaints of chronic low back pain. The physician researched her past pain prescriptions and realized her complaints were consistent with drug-seeking behavior caused by opioid abuse.

   Assign the ICD-10-CM code(s). _____

5. Virgil C.

Virgil was scheduled for his screening colonoscopy, which was performed at the ambulatory surgery center. During the colonoscopy, a sigmoid polyp was removed via the snare technique. He developed hypotension (post-op) that required observation for 24 hours.

a. *Which section of the* ICD-10-CM *Official Guidelines for Coding and Reporting pertain to the*

   sequencing of this primary diagnosis? _____

b. *Assign the ICD-10-CM code(s), sequencing the primary diagnosis first.* _____

6. Mohammed H.

Mohammed was brought to the ED after he passed out in the grocery store. EKG and CT scan of the brain were negative. Laboratory tests were positive for hypoglycemia. He has steroid-induced diabetes caused by long-term use of prednisone for his rheumatoid arthritis.

a. *What is the symptom that required the ED visit?* _____

b. *Assign the ICD-10-CM code(s), sequencing the primary diagnosis first.* _____

7. Tylesa A.

Tylesa presents to the ambulatory surgery unit for acute on chronic tonsillitis, undergoes tonsillectomy and adenoidectomy (T&A), and during post-op develops severe acute postoperative hemorrhage that requires observation after control of bleeding.

Assign the ICD-10-CM code(s), sequencing the primary diagnosis first. _____

8. Mona V.

Mona presented to the physician office with shortness of breath, leg edema, and positive findings of acute systolic congestive heart failure. The patient stopped taking Lasix because of financial hardship. Diagnosis: Acute on chronic CHF caused by underdosing of Lasix.

Assign the ICD-10-CM code(s), sequencing the primary diagnosis first. _____

9. Liam M.

Liam presented to the physician office because of left flank pain. He then was directed to the hospital for x-ray, which revealed left hydronephrosis. Because of severe pain, Liam went directly to the cystoscopy suite for cystoscopy with retrograde pyelogram that revealed a left ureteral calculus.

a. *What diagnosis is reported for the physician office visit?* _____

b. *Assign the ICD-10-CM code(s) for the hospital.* _____

10. Patrick S.

Patrick suffered from left ankle pain after a fall off a swing at the park and went to see Dr. Ramirez, who sent him to the hospital for a left ankle x-ray. X-ray revealed an acute bimalleolar fracture of the ankle. The next day, Patrick underwent an open reduction of the fracture in the ambulatory surgery center. Two weeks later, he presented to Dr. Ramirez for routine aftercare of the fracture for cast change.

a. *Assign the ICD-10-CM code(s) for the first office visit.* _____

b. *Assign the ICD-10-CM code(s) for the outpatient x-ray visit.* _____

c. *Assign the ICD-10-CM code(s) for the ambulatory surgery visit.* _____

d. *Assign the ICD-10-CM external cause code(s).* _____

e. *Assign the ICD-10-CM code(s) for the second visit to Dr. Ramirez.* _____

INTERNET RESEARCH

1. Discover the details of undergoing ambulatory surgery by visiting the following website: www.emedicinehealth.com and search for "outpatient surgery." Read an article about ambulatory surgery preparation, the surgery itself, after surgery, and the synonyms used to reference ambulatory surgery. Identify the documents found in the medical record of an ambulatory surgery patient.

2. An ED visit is one type of outpatient visit. Access the following website: www.livescience .com/strangenews/050526_emergency_visits.html. Determine how many ED visits there are per year. What is one of the primary reasons for these visits? Imagine coding each visit.

3. Many outpatient tests or procedures are covered by Medicare. Policies called National Coverage Determinations (NCDs) and Local Coverage Determinations (LCDs) are available at the Medicare website on their Medicare Coverage Database. These policies provide information for specific tests or services regarding whether or not these services are paid by insurance. Also listed are the ICD-10-CM diagnosis codes that indicate medical necessity for a particular test or service. Access the Medicare website and search the NCD and LCD database for any policy regarding obesity: www.cms.gov/medicare-coverage-database/.

4. Search for the key word "obesity" and choose your geographic location after accessing the Medicare Coverage Database. Which diagnosis code(s) provide medical necessity for treatment of obesity?

5. There are numerous Internet newsletters available for many outpatient settings. Access the website of HCPro (www.hcpro.com) and look at the latest information for the physician office setting. Sign up to receive the free email newsletter.

MEDICAL CODING LAB Remember to use the coding activities at **Medicalcodinglab.com** for extra practice on what you have just learned and to test your knowledge.

CHAPTER 11

ICD-10-PCS Overview and Format

In the health-care setting, different classification systems and nomenclature are used to report procedures depending on the provider and setting of the medical service. Hospitals use the ICD-10-PCS system to collect data, determine payment, and support the electronic health record for all inpatient procedures performed in the United States. ICD-10-PCS was designed to enable each code to have a standard structure and be descriptive yet be flexible enough to accommodate current and future multiple uses of electronically coded data. Chapter 11 in *Conquer Medical Coding* discusses the organization, content, and structure of ICD-10-PCS. The chapter also explains:

- The background and history of ICD-10-PCS and the comparison to ICD-9-CM, Volume 3
- The importance of the *ICD-10-PCS Official Guidelines for Coding and Reporting*
- The conventions used in ICD-10-PCS
- The seven characters of an ICD-10-PCS procedure code
- The basic process of assigning ICD-10-PCS codes
- The online coding resource used to assist in the assignment of accurate ICD-10-PCS codes

CODE IT!

Assign all pertinent ICD-10-PCS codes to the following procedures or diagnostic tests.

1. _____ Percutaneous incision and drainage of left buttock abscess with no drainage device

2. _____ Laparoscopic cholecystectomy

3. _____ Percutaneous, diagnostic thoracentesis for drainage of left pleural effusion

4. _____ Right renal transplantation with donor matched kidney (allogenic) (tissue transplanted from one person to another)

5. _____ Total open right knee replacement with cemented synthetic substitute

6. _____ MR angiography (fluoroscopy) of the left lower extremity arteries with low osmolar contrast

7. _____ Electron beam radiation therapy of the lung

8. _____ Audiovisual motor speech therapy

9. _____ Open low cervical transverse cesarean section

10. _____ Laryngoscopy

MULTIPLE CHOICE

Select the option that best provides the correct code, completes the statement, or answers the question.

1. Debridement of the right lower leg including removal of necrotic muscle using jet lavage is coded as:
   A. OKBS0ZX
   B. OKBS0ZZ
   C. 0KDR0ZZ
   D. 0KDS0ZZ

2. Open reduction and internal fixation of four thoracic rib fractures using titanium plates is coded as:
   A. 0PS204Z
   B. 0PS104Z
   C. 0PS20ZZ
   D. 0PS10ZZ

3. Supracervical hysterectomy in which the uterus was removed through the vaginal opening is coded as:
   A. 0UT97ZL
   B. 0UT90ZL
   C. 0UT47ZZ
   D. 0OB97ZZ

4. Left inguinal hernia repair with synthetic MESH is coded as:
   A. 0WUF0JZ
   B. 0YU61JZ
   C. 0YU50JZ
   D. 0YU60KZ

5. Femoral-femoral artery bypass graft of the left lower leg using venous bypass is coded as:
   A. 041L0ZJ
   B. 041L49H
   C. 041L40AJ
   D. 041L09J

6. Open right axillary lymphadenectomy of the complete chain is coded as:
   A. 07T60ZZ
   B. 07T50ZZ
   C. 07B50ZZ
   D. 07B50ZX

7. Percutaneous bone marrow biopsy from the right iliac crest is coded as:
   A. 07DR3ZX
   B. 07DR0ZX
   C. 07DR3ZZ
   D. 0Q923ZX

8. Open reduction, displaced fracture of the right humeral head is coded as:
   A. 0PSC3ZZ
   B. 2W3AX1Z
   C. 0PSD04Z
   D. 0PSC0ZZ

9. Percutaneous transluminal angioplasty of right radial artery stenosis is coded as:
   A. 037B4ZZ
   B. 03QB3ZZ
   C. 037B3ZZ
   D. 03QB4ZZ

10. Open placement of dual-chamber, rate responsive pacemaker into subcutaneous tissue of the chest wall with leads inserted into the right atrium and ventricle using the percutaneous approach is coded as:
    A. 0JH605Z, 02H63JZ, 02HK3JZ
    B. 0JH636Z, 02H63JZ
    C. 0JH606Z, 02H63JZ, 02HK3JZ
    D. 0JH635Z, 02H63JZ, 02HK3JZ

SHORT ANSWER

Answer the following questions.

1. When coding ICD-10-PCS, it is (always or never) necessary to consult the Alphabetic Index and then proceed to the tables. _____

2. What is the root operation defined as freeing a body part from an abnormal physical constraint by cutting or by the use of force? _____

3. How many codes would be assigned for a resection of a joint with joint replacement? _____

4. Which coding system would the surgeon use to report an inpatient coronary artery bypass graft? _____

5. Materials such as sutures, ligatures, radiological markers, and temporary post-op wound drains (should or should not) be coded separately using ICD-10-PCS device codes. _____

   _____

6. When coding irrigation of a percutaneous nephrostomy tube what is the body system value in the Administration section that would be used? _____

7. ICD-10-PCS denotes which body part as the site that separates upper or lower classifications? _____

   _____

8. Which term in ICD-10-PCS is used to classify a laparoscopic approach? _____

9. Which section of PCS defines procedures in which a diagnostic or therapeutic substance is given to the patient, such as a platelet transfusion? _____

   _____

10. In ICD-10-PCS, this term refers to a series of levels obtained at intervals. _____

CASE STUDIES

1. Farimah G.

> **PREOPERATIVE DIAGNOSIS:** Screening colonoscopy, history of Crohn's disease.
> **POSTOPERATIVE DIAGNOSIS:** Small colonic polyp.
> **PROCEDURE:** Colonoscopy with hot biopsy polypectomy.
> **DESCRIPTION OF PROCEDURE:** Informed consent was obtained for the procedure. The patient was placed in the left lateral decubitus position and sedated with a normal amount of monitored anesthesia care (MAC) sedation. The scope was passed easily into the rectum and was passed up to the level of the cecum. In the sigmoid colon at 15 cm, a 2-mm polyp was seen and removed by hot biopsy polypectomy. The scope was passed to the level of the cecum. The scope was withdrawn from the patient. The patient tolerated the procedure well without complications.

Which root operation would be reported for the polypectomy? Assign the ICD-10-PCS code for

this case. _____

_____

_____

2. Ermano T.

> **PREOPERATIVE DIAGNOSIS:** Urinary frequency.
> **PROCEDURE PERFORMED:** Flexible cystourethroscopy.
> **PROCEDURE:** The patient was placed supine on the operating table and prepped and draped in sterile fashion. Intraurethral Xylocaine was instilled and, after an appropriate length of time, an Olympus flexible cystourethroscope was passed under direct vision. The anterior urethra was normal. The prostatic urethra was patent from the VERU. On cystoscopy, there was grade 2 trabeculation with no evidence of tumors, ulcers, or calculi. The ureteral orifices were visualized with clear efflux bilaterally. The bladder neck was observed with no additional findings. The instrument was withdrawn and there were no additional findings. The patient tolerated the procedure well and left the operating room in satisfactory condition.

Name the operative approach used for this procedure. Assign the ICD-10-PCS code for this case. _____

_____

_____

3. Ralph D.

> **PREOPERATIVE DIAGNOSIS:** Abnormal PSA.
> **PROCEDURE PERFORMED:** Ultrasound-guided prostate biopsies.
> **INDICATIONS:** Ralph is a 68-year-old man with an abnormal PSA of 6.3. His prostate gland is enlarged but smooth.
> **PROCEDURE:** Prostate ultrasound images were obtained in the transverse and longitudinal planes. Total gland volume was 107 cc with a gland length of 64.8 mm. The prostate capsule appears intact. The seminal vesicles are enlarged but symmetric. In the central gland, a large amount of hypertrophy is noted. In the peripheral zone, several small hypoechoic areas are seen. After injection of 10 cc of 1% lidocaine through a spinal needle to the angle of seminal vesicles, six biopsies were taken from each lobe of the prostate. The patient tolerated the procedure well and was returned to the dressing area in stable condition.

Name the operative approach used for this procedure. Assign the ICD-10-PCS code for this case. _____

_____

_____

4. Karyme J.

> **PREOPERATIVE DIAGNOSIS:** Multiparity, desires sterility.
> **OPERATION:** Laparoscopic bilateral tubal ligation.
> **PROCEDURE:** After proper informed consent, the patient was taken to the operating room and placed on the operating table. After adequate induction with general endotracheal anesthesia, she was prepped and draped in the usual sterile fashion. The urinary bladder was drained and a uterine manipulator was placed. A small infraumbilical incision was created with the scalpel blade. The step trocar was inserted without difficulty. A pneumoperitoneum was created once proper placement was confirmed.
> The camera was inserted and detailed visual examination was carried out with the previously mentioned findings. A suprapubic trocar was inserted under direct visualization with care taken to avoid injuring the intra-abdominal contents. The right fallopian tube was traced to its fimbriated end and a Falope ring was applied to the isthmic portion of the tube. Proper placement was confirmed.
> A similar procedure was carried out on the opposite side. Proper placement of both Falope rings was confirmed visually. Photographs were taken. The detailed examination was carried out, searching for endometriosis because of the small amount of blood present. There was no visible endometriosis. The suprapubic trocar was removed under direct visualization and hemostasis was confirmed. The pneumoperitoneum was then reduced and the infraumbilical trocar was removed under direct visualization. Hemostasis was confirmed. The incisions were reapproximated with Vicryl suture in an interrupted fashion. Sterile bandages were applied to the incisions.

Is a Falope ring an extraluminal or intraluminal device? Assign the ICD-10-PCS code for this case. _____

_____

_____

5. Alisa H.

POSTOPERATIVE DIAGNOSIS: Herniated disc left L4–L5 with lumbar radiculopathy.
OPERATIVE PROCEDURE: Left L4–L5 total microdiscectomy.
SPECIMEN: Disc material, intraoperative fluoroscopy was used and intraoperative microdissection was used.
PROCEDURE DESCRIPTION: After the patient was placed prone on the operating table, her back was prepped and draped in the usual manner. A small incision was made slightly paraspinal to the spinous process to the left, and with sharp and blunt dissection lamina and facets of L4 and L5 were exposed. Intraoperative x-rays were used for localization again, and the minimally invasive retractors were placed in position. The laminotomy was performed with the help of Kerrison punches, and ligamentum flavum was removed. A microscope was brought into the field. After extending the laminotomy and medial facetectomy decompressing the lateral recess of the part of the ligamentum, flavum was removed as well. The nerve root was identified and retracted gently without help of cotton paddies. The disc was identified and opened with a #15 blade in a square window shape manner. The discectomy was performed with the help of pituitary rongeurs in various orientations and the disc was irrigated with pressure with a 14-gauge Angiocath and 10-cc syringe. Several large and small fragments of the disc material were removed. No disc was available to pituitary rongeurs and various other instrumentation. The retractors were removed. Hemostasis was confirmed. The nerve root was found to be with compression at the completion of the procedure. The retractors were removed. Fascia was closed with #0 Vicryl. The paraspinal muscle was infiltrated with Marcaine solution. The subcuticular tissue was closed with #3-0 Vicryl, and the skin was closed with Dermabond and Steri-Strips. The patient tolerated the procedure well and was sent to the recovery room in stable condition.

Is L4–L5 lumbar space considered an upper or lower joint? Assign the ICD-10-PCS code for this case. _____

_____

_____

6. Suzanne A.

PREOPERATIVE Diagnosis: Esotropia.
OPERATION: Recession of medial and rectus muscle, bilateral, 4 mm.
PROCEDURE: The patient was taken to the operating room and placed under general anesthesia. Attention was turned to the recession of the right medial rectus muscle. An inferior medial fornix incision was made through the conjunctiva and Tenon's capsule. The medial rectus muscle was then isolated using three successive muscle hooks. The pole test was performed to ensure the entire muscle was hooked. A doubled-armed 6-0 Vicryl was used to suture the muscle with locking bites at each end. The muscle was detached from the globe and the suture was inspected and found to be intact. The muscle was then reattached to the sclera 4 mm posterior to the original insertion site. The conjunctivae were closed using buried interrupted 8-0 Dexon sutures.

How does ICD-10-PCS classify the body part for the medial and rectus muscle of the eye? Assign the ICD-10-PCS code for this case. _____

_____

_____

7. Neema N.

PREOPERATIVE DIAGNOSIS: Mammographic abnormality of the left breast.
PROCEDURE: Needle-localized left excisional breast biopsy.
OPERATION: After adequate sedation was achieved, the patient's left breast was prepped with Betadine and draped in a sterile fashion. A curvilinear incision, just inferior to the localizing needle, was made with a knife. Dissection was carried down bluntly. An Allis clamp was then placed on the specimen and sharp dissection carried around the perimeter, providing a generous core of tissue surrounding the top of the localizing needle. The specimen was then radiographed with the findings previously noted. The base of the cavity was then packed with a dry sponge. Pressure was held for several minutes. Cautery was required to obtain hemostasis, which was adequate at the completion of the procedure. Deep interrupted stitches of 3-0 Vicryl were placed, followed by a running subcuticular stitch of 4-0 Vicryl. Mastisol, Steri-Strips, Adaptic, and gauze were then placed and taped securely.

How many ICD-10-PCS codes would be assigned if a biopsy was completed on both breasts? Assign the ICD-10-PCS code for this case. _____

_____

_____

8. Timothy D.

PREOPERATIVE and **POSTOPERATIVE DIAGNOSIS:** Closed displaced right second metacarpal neck fracture.
OPERATION: Open reduction internal fixation right metacarpal neck fracture.
PROCEDURE: A well-padded tourniquet was placed on the right upper arm and the right upper extremity was prepped and draped in sterile orthopedic fashion. Attempts were initially made for closed reduction and pinning of the fracture. This was attempted multiple times from a retrograde and anagrade fashion without success. A 3-cm incision was then made directly over the metacarpal head and fracture. Sharp dissection was carried out through the skin and subcutaneous tissue. The extensor tendon was then identified and slid ulnarly. A dent was made in the capsule. The fracture was identified and reduced. From a proximal to distal fashion, a 0.062 K-wire was introduced into the metacarpal shaft, across the fracture and into the metacarpal head. It was found to be stable. Under AP, lateral, and oblique image intensification, the hardware was in good position and not penetrating the joint. It was then cut beneath the skin. All open wounds were then irrigated. The two stab wounds that had been made prior were closed with interrupted 4-0 nylon. The rent in the capsule was closed with figure-of-eight-0-Vicryl and then the skin was closed with 4-0 nylon.

Review the operative report and identify the specific device used to reduce the fracture. Assign the ICD-10-PCS procedure code for the open reduction. _____

_____

_____

9. Paul V.

> **PROCEDURE:**
> 1. #8 French PTCI sheath was placed in the right femoral artery in the usual manner.
> 2. Single vessel angiography was performed with a #8 French FL4 guiding catheter.
> 3. Balloon angioplasty was performed of the distal circumflex marginal with a 2.0 x 20 mm balloon.
> 4. Intracoronary stenting with 2.5 x 8 mm Tristar drug-eluting stents were placed in tandem across the stenosed area.
>
> Once guiding shots were obtained, a 0.014 Allstar 190-cm length wire was passed through the virtually 100% occluded circumflex marginal into the distal vessel. The vessel was then dilated with a 2.0 x 20 mm Crossail balloon once, maximum 1 minute, maximum 8 bars. Then, a 2.5 x 8 mm Tristar stent was deployed across the lesion at 10 bars x 1 minute. At this point, the stenosis appeared to be widely dilated; however, there was a hazy segment perhaps with some contrast hangup just distal to the stent. It was felt this may be a dissection; a second 2.5 x 8 mm Tristar stent was deployed across this area, somewhat overlapping the first stent but extending distally at 8 bars x 1 minute. The stent balloon was withdrawn a few millimeters and then redilated 10 bars x 30 seconds.
>
> Coronary angiography then revealed the stenosis to be reduced from virtually 100% to –5%. There was TIMI III flow at the conclusion with good flow in the distal vessel. The previously noted contrast, "hangup," was now not seen. The patient had no chest pain, EKG was at base-line, and he was hemodynamically stable at the conclusion of the case.
>
> **CONCLUSION:** Successful stenting of the distal circumflex marginal coronary artery.

Do the number of stents inserted impact the ICD-10-CM code assignment? Assign the ICD-10-PCS code for this case. _____

_____

_____

10. Bobby E.

> **POSTOPERATIVE DIAGNOSIS:** A 12-year-old patient with sleep apnea secondary to hypertrophic tonsils and adenoids.
> **OPERATION:** Tonsillectomy and adenoidectomy (T&A).
> **PROCEDURE:** After preanesthesia with fentanyl, Robinul, and Inapsine, the patient was brought to the operating room (OR) and placed in the usual supine position. After satisfactory general endotracheal anesthesia was obtained, a medium Crowe-Davis mouth gag was inserted. The adenoids were palpated and felt to be obstructing the nasopharynx and removed using a curettage technique. The tonsils were then removed using the dissection snare technique. Hemostasis in both cases was obtained with tonsil balls soaked in bismuth subgallate, as well as Bovie coagulum. Blood loss was 20 cc. The patient tolerated the procedure well and returned to recovery in good condition.

Assign the ICD-10-PCS code(s) for this case. _____

_____

MEDICAL CODING LAB Remember to use the coding activities at **Medicalcodinglab.com** for extra practice on what you have just learned and to test your knowledge.

CHAPTER 12

CPT Basics

The Common Procedural Terminology (CPT) code set is based on the various types of professional services performed by physicians and other health-care professionals such as physician's assistants; nurses; physical, occupational, and speech therapists; chiropractors; and dietitians. CPT codes cover thousands of professional services, from office visits to surgery, radiology, laboratory and pathology, anesthesiology, and other medical procedures. Chapter 12 in *Conquer Medical Coding* introduces the format of the CPT manual and explains procedural coding fundamentals and guidelines. In addition to explaining the nine steps to accurately assign CPT codes and append appropriate modifiers, the chapter covers:

- The uses of data collected from health-care claims
- The medical settings in which CPT is used
- The meaning of the symbols, format, and punctuation used in CPT
- The purpose and use of CPT modifiers and the distinction among CPT professional, HCPCS, and facility modifiers
- CPT coding resources and references
- When an unlisted code is required
- The purpose and parts of a special report

CODE IT!

Assign all pertinent CPT codes to the following procedures.

1. _____ Percutaneous needle core biopsy of the breast

2. _____ Injection carpal tunnel ligament

3. _____ Open biopsy, vertebral body, thoracic

4. _____ Removal of anal seton

With the use of the CPT section guidelines, identify the following unlisted procedure codes.

5. _____ Medicine: Special dermatological service

6. _____ Surgery–Digestive: Unlisted laparoscopy procedure, biliary tract

Assign the most appropriate modifier to each of the following statements.

7. _____ Surgeon administers a regional Bier block because of ruptured sutures.

8. _____ Patient hemorrhaged heavily during surgery; procedure took twice as long as is typically required.

9. _____ Surgeon repairs the flexor tendon of the right foot and excises a ganglion on the right fourth toe.

10. _____ During an operation, a thoracic surgeon provides surgical access to the spine while an orthopedist performs a spinal fusion.

MULTIPLE CHOICE

Select the option that best completes the statement or answers the question.

1. Which of the following identifies codes that have been revised?
   A. ★
   B. ⊃
   C. ⁄
   D. ▲

2. Anesthesia services are organized by:
   A. Place of service
   B. Type of procedure
   C. Body site
   D. Body system

3. A service not included in the surgery package is:
   A. Separate procedures
   B. Routine follow-up from a surgical hysteroscopy
   C. Office visit where decision for surgery was made
   D. Pre-op appointment the day before the scheduled surgery

4. A patient is on vacation out of state and breaks her left ankle. The patient sees a doctor there who sets the fracture. The patient returns home several days later and will follow up with a local physician. The out-of-state physician will report which modifier?
   A. −55
   B. −57
   C. −56
   D. −54

5. A special report is required in which of the following circumstances?
   A. Unlisted procedure code
   B. Submitting modifier −22
   C. Submitting modifier −59
   D. All of the above

6. The patient is returned to the operating room 3 hours after surgery for a related procedure; service is being billed by a hospital outpatient facility. Which modifier applies?
   A. −51
   B. −78
   C. −76
   D. −58

7. A radiologist who is not employed by the hospital provides the interpreting and reporting for all x-rays taken at the hospital. Which modifier is used to reflect her services?
   A. −51
   B. −59
   C. −No modifier needed
   D. −26

8. A(n) _____ procedure code is used when there is no other designated code to describe a procedure or service.
   A. Unlisted
   B. Separate
   C. HCPCS
   D. Category III

9. When you see the ▲ symbol in front of a code, what do you know about the code?
   A. It's a new code
   B. It's a physician-only code
   C. It's an add-on code
   D. It's a revised code

10. Identify the main term from this statement: "Sinus endoscopy with concha bullosa resection."
    A. Resection
    B. Endoscopy
    C. Sinus
    D. Concha bullosa

SHORT ANSWER

Answer the following questions.

1. List two modifiers (not physical status modifiers) that describe anesthesia services. _____

_____

2. Name three instances in which the −51 modifier is not appropriate to append. _____

_____

_____

3. Which organization developed and maintains CPT codes and guidelines? _____

_____

4. Using CPT, refer to the notes immediately preceding the code 45300 and to the code series 45300–45378 and answer this question: If a colonoscopy is incomplete due to unforeseen circumstances, but full preparation for the procedure has been done, which modifier should be used? _____

_____

5. When are updated CPT codes released? As of what annual date do they go into effect? _____

_____

6. The + symbol indicates that this is a(n) _____ code.

7. The ⊘ symbol indicates that the _____ modifier does not apply.

8. When a procedure is marked "separate procedure," you can bill for it if it was _____ _____, or in a(n) _____, or _____ of any other related service provided.

9. A CPT code can be located in the index by looking for the _____ or service performed; _____ for which the patient is being treated; _____, _____, _____ site; or _____.

10. In the following list, label each entry as a section, procedure, heading, subcategory, or subsection.

    a. Excision _____

    b. Surgery _____

    c. Salivary gland and ducts _____

    d. Excision of submandibular gland _____

    e. Digestive _____

CASE STUDIES

1. Andrew F.

   Andrew fractured his tibia in Vermont while skiing. The surgery to repair the tibia was performed in Vermont. Andrew was so anxious to get back home that he left 2 days after surgery to be seen by his own orthopedist, who did all of the follow-up care.

   *Which modifier will the provider at home report?*_____

2. Celia H.

   Celia previously had two abnormal Pap smears and is scheduled for biopsy. She also has breakthrough bleeding in between menstrual cycles and will have endometrial sampling performed. Celia is seen in the GYN office for a colposcopy and biopsy of the cervix at the 7 o'clock position and endometrial sampling. The physician instructs the billing office to report codes 57454 and 58100.

   Are these services being correctly coded and reported? How do you know? _____

   _____

   _____

3. Sara K.

   Sara, a 45-year-old female, is seen at a general surgery office for treatment of fibroadenomas of the right breast. The two masses are being monitored and have grown slightly in size, one in the upper left quadrant and the second in the lower left quadrant. Sara elects to have cryoablation performed as opposed to a lumpectomy. Using ultrasound to guide, the physician inserts the cryoprobe into the center of the first lesion, forming an iceball. The cryoprobe is then inserted into the second tumor under ultrasound guidance until an iceball forms.

   Assign the correct CPT code(s) for this encounter. _____

   _____

4. Oko Z.

   An orthopedist examines Oko and determines that he has a ruptured C3–C4 intervertebral disk with severe radiating pain to the right arm. The orthopedist fully examines Oko's history, performs x-rays, and completes a physical. After reviewing the films, the orthopedist requests that a neurologist perform the actual surgery because the orthopedist does not routinely perform surgery on the cervical spine.

   The orthopedist will submit the surgical code for this procedure along with which modifier? _____

   _____

5. Kirsten O.

Kirsten is seen in the office for complaints of congestion, fever, and sinus headache for 4 consecutive days. She is examined by the nurse practitioner and diagnosed with acute rhinosinusitis. She orders an IgE blood test since the patient has recurrent chronic rhinosinusitis. The in-house phlebotomist draws the blood. The nurse practitioner prescribes an antibiotic and administers a steroid shot in the hip. The office visit is billed with 99213.

a. *What other service should be billed and why can it be reported separately?* _____

_____

b. *How is this reported?* _____

c. *Is a modifier required? If so, on which code?* _____

_____

6. Lacey N.

Lacey, a 4-year-old girl, is seen in the urgent care center for persistent dry cough and increasing shortness of breath for the last 24 hours. She is examined and her lungs sound raspy. A chest x-ray is performed, frontal and lateral view. Films are reviewed on-site by a physician who is not employed by the center. There is no congestion or fluid build-up in her lungs. Lacey is diagnosed with an acute asthma attack and given an inhalation nebulizer treatment and IV corticosteroids.

a. *What is the place of service (POS) for this encounter?* _____

_____

b. *Which services are reportable (aside from the E/M) service discussed in Chapter 13 of this text)?* _____

_____

_____

c. *Assign the procedure codes for the facility.* _____

7. Carl U.

Carl was taken to the ED by ambulance after his wife heard a thud upstairs and found him unconscious. The patient does not remember tripping, falling, or losing consciousness. Upon arrival, Carl is evaluated with a thorough history and examination. He is awake and oriented but his BP is elevated and he has a slight tremor of his right hand. EKG was normal. Carotid ultrasound Doppler study was performed on both carotid arteries and there was no evidence of stenosis or blockage.

a. *What is the POS?* _____

_____

b. *Assign the procedure codes for the facility (aside from E/M service):* _____

_____

8. Amanda P.

Amanda is seen in the dermatology office for an annual skin examination. She has numerous moles on her neck and back and is concerned about cancer. She thinks one of them is getting larger. A complete physical skin examination is performed. Amanda is counseled on the need to perform monthly self-examinations for new or changing moles.

What Category II code(s) is reported to demonstrate this preventive intervention was carried out to track

quality patient care? _____

_____

9. Rasalan S.

Rasalan, a 40-year-old female patient, desires sterilization and elects to proceed with a tubal occlusion procedure in the OB/GYN office. Rasalan is taken to the minor procedure room and the anesthetist administers the IV Versed for conscious sedation. The physician begins the procedure by inserting the hysteroscope into the vagina and then inserts a cannula into the right fallopian os and places the occlusion device. Attention is turned to the left fallopian tube os. The opening cannot be located after several attempts to visualize and probe the opening. The physician stops looking and the procedure ends. The physician will schedule the patient for outpatient surgery next week to occlude the left fallopian tube laparoscopically with a Hulka clip.

a. *What is the procedure code?* _____

b. *Is this considered a discontinued procedure or a reduced service?*_____

_____

c. *What modifier(s) are reported?* _____

d. *Can this procedure be reported with conscious sedation? If so, by whom?* _____

_____

10. Lee-Ann B.

Lee-Ann, a coder working in a physician office, is responsible for updating the office encounter form, in-house lab requisitions, and office computer system. She has to look for changes to diagnosis and procedure codes and keep these current at all times.

a. *How often are diagnosis codes updated?* _____

b. *How often are CPT codes updated?* _____

c. *For changes to CPT codes, where would she look to find these changes?* _____

_____

INTERNET RESEARCH

1. a. Visit the website of the American Medical Association at www.ama-assn.org. Click on the *Resources* heading. Scroll toward the bottom and select *CPT Products and Services* followed by *About CPT*. Read the information on the CPT process, and report on how new CPT codes are approved.
   b. Assume that you are working as a coder. Based on the update schedule for Category III codes, what advice would you provide about when to update your resources for selecting these codes?
2. Medical societies such as the American Academy of Family Physicians offer Internet tools to support their coding. Go to www.aafp.org, and locate this year's CPT code updates. Prepare a report on other related information that you consider valuable from this website.
3. Visit the U.S. Preventive Services Task Force website at www.uspreventiveservicestaskforce .org/uspstf/uspsabrecs.htm and list three services from the A and B Recommendations that may be reported with modifier −33.

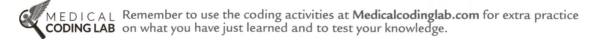 MEDICAL CODING LAB Remember to use the coding activities at **Medicalcodinglab.com** for extra practice on what you have just learned and to test your knowledge.

CHAPTER 13

CPT: Evaluation and Management Codes

Chapter 13 in *Conquer Medical Coding* introduces coding for evaluation and management (E/M) services. These services represent the physician's evaluation of a patient's condition and management of a patient's care. The time, effort, and training required to perform them varies widely according to the situation. Because the services provided vary so widely, many are paid on a scale that reflects time, effort, and complexity. Recall that working with E/M codes requires an understanding of the structure of the E/M section. You can locate the correct code range in the E/M categories and then pick the correct code while studying and answering the following standard set of five questions:

1. Who is the patient?
2. What is the place of service?
3. What is the patient's status?
4. What type of service is being provided?
5. What level of service is being provided?

In addition to describing the organization of the CPT E/M section and the process used to determine the level of service for E/M coding, Chapter 13 explains:

- The difference between new and established patients in CPT terms
- The three key components that determine the level of service and the levels of each component
- The factors that are important in assigning critical care codes
- Observation and standby services
- The correct application of the rules and exceptions for each category of service

CODE IT!

Assign all pertinent CPT codes to the following diagnoses or conditions.

1. _____ Code for 40 minutes of critical care services provided by a physician for an eighteen month old during transport.

2. _____ Code for initial observation care provided at the hospital with a detailed history, comprehensive examination, and moderate medical decision making (MD).

3. _____ An established patient is seen in the office and the physician documented a detailed examination and low MDM. Code for the visit.

4. _____ A neonatologist was called to treat a critically ill neonate in the intensive care unit. The child had just arrived in the hospital. Code for the neonatologist's services.

5. _____ Code for the non-face-to-face services provided by a patient's supervising physician while the patient was under the care of a home health agency. The physician spent 20 minutes on the patient during that month.

6. _____ This physician had not seen his patient in 4 years. He provided a detailed history, a detailed examination, with low medical decision making (MDM). What code should be used?

7. _____ After a motor vehicle accident (MVA), an injured passenger is taken by ambulance to the emergency department (ED). The ED physician provides a detailed history and examination and moderate MDM.

8. _____ A cardiologist is asked for her opinion regarding an inpatient's chest pain. The history is expanded problem focused (EPF), the examination is detailed, and the MDM is low. The cardiologist documents his findings in the patient's chart. What code should be used?

9. _____ A patient's uncle suggests he see a thoracic surgeon for a second opinion on the need for surgery. The patient has never seen this physician before. Is this a new patient code or a consultation code?

10. _____ For the month of November, a physician has spent 20 minutes discussing care plans with the hospice nurse for his patient who is under hospice care. What code should the physician report?

MULTIPLE CHOICE

Select the option that best provides the correct code, completes the statement, or answers the question.

1. During a new patient visit for an 84-year-old male whose voice is hoarse, the patient has difficulty breathing. The history was detailed, examination was detailed, and MDM was low. What is the correct way to code this situation?
   A. 99203
   B. 99204
   C. 99202
   D. 99214

2. A patient is admitted to the hospital with pancreatitis. The physician provided initial hospital care with a detailed history, comprehensive examination, and high MDM. What is the correct way to code this situation?
   A. 99203
   B. 99221
   C. 99233
   D. 99218

3. A patient goes to the ED via ambulance after an MVA with moderate injuries. The ED physician performs a detailed history and examination and moderate MDM. What is the correct way to code this situation?
   A. 99284
   B. 99282
   C. 99243
   D. 99244

4. An inpatient is seen in follow up by the attending physician 5 days after admission. The physician performs a problem focused (PF) history, EPF examination, and moderate MDM. What is the correct way to code this situation?
   A. 99241
   B. 99212
   C. 99233
   D. 99232

5. The patient returns to the office for continued cold-like symptoms. She complains of constant runny nose, has an escalated cough, and has a fever. The patient states she is unable to work. The physician performs a detailed examination, detailed history, and low MDM. What is the correct way to code this situation?
   A. 99214
   B. 99213
   C. 99204
   D. 99212

6. An internal medicine physician has admitted a patient to the hospital and requests that a cardiologist provide an opinion on the patient's chest pain. The cardiologist reviews the patient's chart, as well as all diagnostic tests and monitoring. The patient got good relief of her chest pain with Maalox. The MDM was straightforward, EPF history was obtained, and the examination was detailed. The cardiologist reported his findings in the shared medical record. What is the correct way to code this situation?
   A. 99242
   B. 99243
   C. 99252
   D. 99251

7. An established patient has a reaction to insulin and comes to the office. The physician performs an EPF examination, PF history, and moderate MDM. The patient is kept for several hours for observation and monitoring. The doctor spends a total of 2 hours with the patient. What is the correct way to code this situation?
   A. 99213, 99354, 99355x2
   B. 99214, 99218
   C. 99214, 99354, 99355x2
   D. 99213, 99354, 99355

8. A 12-year-old is seen in the office by his family practitioner of 5 years. He sustained a laceration to his arm after falling off his skateboard. The physician did a 9.5-cm layered closure of the arm (12034). The patient mentions he has begun to develop acne and is very self-conscious; he has also developed an odd rash on his leg. The physician performs an EPF history, EPF examination of the face and leg, and advises the patient to wash his face with soap and water twice a day and apply astringent for straightforward (SF) MDM. What is the correct way to code for the E/M service?
   A. 99201
   B. 99213–25
   C. 99212
   D. E/M not reportable

9. An inpatient female is seen on the physician's hospital rounds. The physician performs a PF history and examination. What is the correct way to code this situation?
   A. Not a reportable service (no MDM was documented)
   B. 99212
   C. 99231
   D. 99238

10. A new patient visit is held for a 14-year-old with a 4-day history of lower abdominal pain, with occasional vomiting but no fever. The physician performs a detailed history and examination, as well as a moderate MDM. The patient tells the physician she is sexually active but has not missed any periods over the past year. The physician counsels the patient on the prevention of sexual diseases for 35 minutes. The total visit was 60 minutes. What is the correct way to code this situation?
    A. 99205
    B. 99203
    C. 99204
    D. 99384

SHORT ANSWER

Answer the following questions.

1. When can time be the dominant factor in determining the level of service? _____

_____

_____

2. Explain the roll-up rule._____

_____

_____

3. Explain the significance of the statement that "the lowest key component controls the level of service."_____

_____

_____

4. A patient moves from New York to South Carolina and sees his new physician for his many complex medical problems. The day before his appointment, the physician spends 45 minutes reviewing the patient's extensive medical records. The physician tells his billing staff that he cannot report the chart review services because he did that work the day before the appointment. Is the physician correct? Explain your answer. _____

_____

_____

5. There are two types of care plan oversight services. What differentiates them? _____

_____

_____

6. The statement "a physician cannot report a consultation code if he or she provided treatment to the patient during the visit" represents what consultation concept? _____

_____

_____

7. What is the 15-minute rule, and what codes use this rule? _____

_____

_____

8. After providing the key components of an E/M service, the physician spent 1 hour counseling the mother and the patient regarding diabetes, diet, and lifestyle changes. Total visit time was 1 hour, 15 minutes. What code should be reported? _____

_____

_____

9. A patient was admitted to the hospital at 11 p.m. Tuesday by the resident. The patient's attending physician sees the patient on Wednesday morning. What range of codes will the attending physician report? _____

_____

10. Provide the code for 1 hour of inpatient pediatric critical care._____

CASE STUDIES

1. Lorena O.

   In reviewing documentation for an E/M service, Lorena, a coder, downcoded the level of service because there was no evidence that one of the E/M contributory components was provided. Lorena explained that she had been taught that at least one of the contributory components has to be documented.

   Is Lorena correct? How would you use this chapter to explain to Lorena why she is or is not

   correct? _____

   _____

   _____

2. Lorena O.

   After reviewing the physician's documentation related to MDM, Lorena the coder noted that the patient had three diagnoses (multiple); one laboratory test was ordered (limited) and the risk level was low.

   What would be the complexity of MDM? _____

   _____

3. Lidia V.

   Lidia, a new patient, is seen today for eczema. It started last week but is now causing her left eye to swell and she is having trouble sleeping. The eczema started on her neck and is now on her face. She currently takes Singulair and albuterol as needed. She is allergic to peanuts. Her diagnosis is atopic dermatitis flare. She will now use Triaminicin cream and Benadryl and should call the office if there is no improvement in 5 days. The history is detailed, the examination is EPF, and MDM is low.

   What is the code for this encounter? _____

   _____

4. Ty W.

   Ty is critically injured and in shock after an MVA while on his motorcycle. He is taken to the ED where the ED physician provides critical care for one hour to stabilize Ty's respiratory failure and life-threatening low blood pressure (BP). He stabilizes, but 2 hours later his BP again drops to 70 over 50 and his breathing is labored. The physician spends another hour to stabilize Ty.

   How should the ED physician code for her services? _____

   _____

5. Chet B.

After several unending snowstorms, Chet, a 60-year-old man, complains of chest pain and sees his family doctor. His symptoms do not appear to be cardiac related (he always eats chili peppers before going out to shovel) but because of the severity of his pain and his blood work results he is admitted to the hospital. While there (and complaining bitterly about being there), Chet again has chest pain (no chili peppers). His attending family doctor requests a cardiologist to evaluate his patient's chest pain. The cardiologist reviews the chart, as well as all diagnostic tests and monitoring. The MDM was straightforward, the history was EPF, and the examination was detailed. The cardiologist reported his findings in the shared medical record.

What is the code for the service(s) provided in this encounter? _____

_____

6. Charlaine I.

Charlaine, a 62-year-old woman, presents to her internist's office for her annual physical. She has had type 2 diabetes for most of her adult life and has recently developed angina. Her physician provides a comprehensive history and examination as part of her preventive medicine visit. She is counseled regarding exercise, diet, and injury prevention, particularly to her lower extremities. Additionally, a history, examination, and MDM are provided because of the new development of angina. The history and examination are EPF, and the MDM is low.

What is the code for the service(s) provided in this encounter? _____

_____

7. Bolton E.

Bolton was seen 1 year ago for Lyme disease and given treatment for 28 days. He is here today for follow up and has improved; however, he has developed a persistent knee effusion. He will start on Naprosyn to treat the knee infusion. The history is detailed, the examination is EPF, and MDM is moderate.

How should the coder report this encounter? _____

_____

8. Augustus G.

Augustus is 9 months old and presents for follow up regarding his vomiting and difficulty sleeping. In his last visit, his formula was changed to see if his condition would improve. He is not vomiting as much and is sleeping better. His mother states he passes a lot of gas. His weight is stable and the physician discusses the risks and benefits of medication for fussiness. The history is PF, the examination is EPF, and MDM is low. The visit lasts a total of 25 minutes, during which the physician spent 10 minutes discussing the patient's fussiness and medication issues.

What is the code for this encounter? _____

_____

9. Shontel W.

A gastroenterologist is asked for her opinion on a 23-year-old inpatient's radiating abdominal pain. The patient, Shontel, was admitted for fracture care of the right shoulder but shortly after admission complained of abdominal pain. The gastroenterologist evaluated the patient and ordered laboratory studies and an x-ray, which did not indicate any injury or disease. Her history and examination were detailed and MDM was moderate. The visit was documented in the patient's chart. The gastroenterologist will follow up with the patient in 2 days.

What is the code for the gastroenterologist? _____

_____

10. Shontel W.

In the follow-up visit at the hospital, Shontel indicated she no longer had any abdominal pain and was fine. The gastroenterologist did a PF history and examination.

What is the code for this encounter? _____

INTERNET RESARCH

1. Visit the following Medicare site that answers frequently asked questions (FAQs) about E/M coding: www.connecticutmedicare.com (On this site, select Resources/Tools, then Medicare FAQs, and scroll down to Evaluation and Management [E/M] services.) Visit the site and report on the types of topics that are discussed.
2. The CMS website has a frequently asked questions FAQs section for the TCM codes. Go to www.cms.gov and type "transitional care management" into the search box. A drop-down menu will offer you a FAQ option. Review these FAQs for help with this coding area.
3. Acronyms are important in medical documentation and particularly in E/M coding. Review the following sites for assistance in finding acronyms:
www.medilexicon.com
www.en.wikipedia.org/wiki/list_of_medical_abbreviations
You can also search for "medical acronyms" with any search engine and find the site that works best for you.

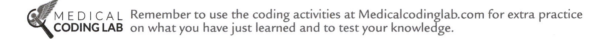 Remember to use the coding activities at Medicalcodinglab.com for extra practice on what you have just learned and to test your knowledge.

CHAPTER 14

CPT: Evaluation and Management Auditing

Payers insist on objective verifiable assessments of evaluation and management (E/M) levels; therefore, rules have been established to quantify these services. Following the rules permits coders, auditors, reviewers, and carriers to decide whether the E/M service a physician has reported is accurately supported by what he or she has documented. This validation in turn provides verification of the reimbursement level for the service. It is most common that physicians will select the E/M level of service (LOS) for each patient encounter. Chapter 14 in *Conquer Medical Coding* explains the process that allows the coder or the auditor to verify that the documentation meets the LOS chosen. In addition, the chapter explains the following information:

- The origin and purpose of documentation guidelines
- How documentation translates into a level of E/M service
- The differences between the 1995 and the 1997 documentation guidelines
- The code for E/M services from physician documentation, and how to use the 1995 documentation guidelines and the 1997 multispecialty and single-specialty documentation guidelines
- The purpose of the audit process
- The tools used for auditing E/M services
- How to successfully complete an audit form from documentation
- How to identify the audit pitfalls of an electronic medical record system

CODE IT!

Supply the correct codes or levels for the following.

1. _____ The new patient has left shoulder pain for 2 weeks caused by a fall. What is the history of present illness (HPI) level.

2. _____ The physician reviewed the patient's respiratory, cardiovascular, and musculoskeletal system. What is the review of systems (ROS) level?

3. _____ The physician documented the patient's past, family, and social history (PFSH). What is the level of PFSH?

4. _____ What code represents the level of history for this new patient based on the 1995 guidelines?

5. _____ The physician examined the patient's musculoskeletal, cardiovascular, gastrointestinal (GI), and integumentary systems. What code represents the level of the examination based on the 1995 guidelines?

6. _____ The physician documented a new problem with no additional workup planned. What is the medical decision making (MDM) level for diagnoses and management options?

7. _____ An x-ray was ordered. What is the MDM level for data review?

8. _____ The risk was for a presenting problem of an acute uncomplicated injury. What is the MDM level for overall risk?

9. _____ Based on the previous three factors, what code represents the level of MDM?

10. _____ Based on the three key components determined in the previous questions, what is the code for this new patient?

MULTIPLE CHOICE

Select the option that best completes the statement or answers the question.

1. A patient presents to his physician's office for headache and dizziness. The patient had been seen 3 months ago for his annual physical, and no problems had been noted. The patient had not fallen or in any way injured his head, but the problem had started about 2 weeks ago after he had received the flu vaccine. The dizziness is worse in the morning. The patient denies any muscle aches or respiratory problems, and has no palpitations, but states that his vision is sometimes blurry. He states that there is no family history of neurological illness that he knows of. What is the level of history?
   A. Detailed
   B. Comprehensive
   C. Problem focused (PF)
   D. Expanded problem focused (EPF)

2. Dr. Smith's patient developed a cardiac arrhythmia after her admission to the hospital for an acute asthma attack. Dr. Smith asked a cardiologist to see the patient and give his opinion on whether the arrhythmia was related to the asthma or to another problem. The cardiologist saw the patient and recorded the encounter in the hospital chart. The cardiologist examined the cardiovascular, respiratory, and digestive systems. The history was detailed, and the MDM was moderate. Based on the 1995 guidelines, which code did the cardiologist report?
   A. 99243
   B. 99252
   C. 99254
   D. 99253

3. The physician documented a patient's diagnosis as right lower quadrant abdominal pain with a question of a possible ulcer or a bowel obstruction. The physician ordered blood work and a barium swallow. She plans to review the results of both tests and may schedule surgery or further tests based on the findings. What service does the preceding information represent?
   A. History
   B. Examination
   C. MDM
   D. None of the above

4. An established patient was having abdominal pain and made an appointment to see her internist. On the day of the appointment, she acknowledged eating too many sweets, which could complicate her diabetes and cause the stomach pain, but she was also feeling very lethargic. No PFSH was documented in the patient's chart; the physician examined her

digestive system and documented her blood pressure (BP), pulse, and weight. The assessment and plan noted diabetes and stomach pain for the diagnoses. The physician ordered blood work and an x-ray, and the overall risk was noted as moderate based on the presenting problem. What is the LOS for this visit based on the 1995 documentation guidelines?
A. 99213
B. 99214
C. 99203
D. Do not report this service; only two key components were documented.

5. A physician documented duration, context, and location in the HPI. She also reviewed three systems and past and family history. The physician examined three organ systems, and her documentation showed a low level of MDM. The services were provided to an established patient. What is the LOS?
A. 99212
B. 99213
C. 99214
D. 99215

6. What would the LOS be if the patient in Question 5 was a new patient?
A. 99201
B. 99202
C. 99203
D. 99204

7. Using the 1997 musculoskeletal examination guidelines, determine the LOS of the following examination: Patient's BP is 142/80; pulse is 78; weight is 168. There is no swelling of the neck nodes; the patient's gait is normal. There is no asymmetry in the legs, but the patient has limited range of motion in both legs.
A. PF
B. EPF
C. Detailed
D. Comprehensive

8. Using the 1997 general multisystem examination guidelines, determine the LOS based on the same documentation as in Question 7.
A. PF
B. EPF
C. Detailed
D. Comprehensive

9. For a ROS, a physician documented GI, neurological, cardiovascular, respiratory, and musculoskeletal. She then indicated "all others negative." How do the documentation guidelines address this type of notation and its relation to the level of the ROS?
A. "All others negative" is not allowed and cannot apply to the ROS.
B. The only way to reach a complete level of ROS is by documenting 10 systems.
C. A notation indicating that all other systems are negative is permissible for the complete level of ROS.
D. The physician must document at least eight systems to allow for the use of "all others negative."

10. Why does CMS consider deliberate downcoding of services fraudulent?
A. Because the physician will be reimbursed at a higher rate
B. Because it is seen as an intent to have patients use the physician's services more often
C. Because the physician will be allowed to bill the patient more often
D. None of the above

SHORT ANSWER

Answer the following questions.

1. Why are there two sets of documentation guidelines? _____

    _____

    _____

2. If a patient is injured because of a fall from a ladder, what element of the history is indicated?

    _____

    _____

3. Is the description of four or more elements or the status of at least three chronic or inactive conditions allowed as an example of the extended level of HPI? _____

    _____

4. Is the rule determined in Question 3 appropriate to the 1995 or 1997 guidelines, or to both?

    _____

    _____

5. The use of the phrase "all others are negative" is found in what key component of the documentation guidelines (DG)? _____

    _____

6. What element of the history key component is considered problematic to providers who report comprehensive levels of service? _____

    _____

7. PFSH has an unusual criterion related to what is considered a complete PFSH. What is that criterion? _____

    _____

8. Should abnormal findings in the affected body area be documented? _____

    _____

9. Is it sufficient to document eight organ systems for a comprehensive level general multisystem examination? _____

    _____

10. What is another term for the risk of significant complications, morbidity, or mortality? _____

    _____

CASE STUDIES

1. Irina S.

> **CHIEF COMPLAINT:** Sinus headache.
> **HPI:** Irina is here because she has had sinus headaches for 2 weeks with green nasal discharge and a productive cough. Patient was last seen 1 year ago for sinus infection.
> **ROS:** There is some ear pain but no breathing difficulties.
> **MEDICATIONS:** Nasacort twice a day.
> **EXAMINATION:** No wheezing, no skin rash; eyes are clear; some fluid in her ears.
> **MDM:** Sinus infection, place on azithromycin. Patient should phone if infection does not resolve by next week.

What E/M code should be reported for this patient, using the 1995 DG? _____

_____

2. Marcus R.

Office Note

> **CHIEF COMPLAINT:** Upper abdominal pain.
> **HPI:** Patient is a 70-year-old male with severe upper abdominal pain that began at 9 p.m. last night. He was last seen 2 years ago. The patient has no shortness of breath and was not exerting himself when the pain started. The patient has had some difficulty with swallowing for the past year.
> **ROS:** Back pain, some visual blurring occasionally, no allergies.
> **PAST MEDICAL HISTORY (PMH):** Bladder carcinoma.
> **PAST SURGICAL HISTORY (PSH):** Hernia repair.
> **MEDICATIONS:** None.
> **SOCIAL HISTORY (SH):** Married, does not smoke.
> **FAMILY HISTORY (FH):** None for GI disease.
> **EXAMINATION:** Weight is 225, BP is 160/80, pulse is 92; lungs are clear to auscultation; cardiovascular shows a normal rate and rhythm; abdomen is positive for bowel sounds and some tenderness.
> **MDM:** Abdominal pain, dysphagia secondary to reflux and stricture formation. Rule out gastroparesis. Schedule for esophagogastroduodenoscopy (EGD).

Provide the E/M codes to be reported for this patient, using both the 1995 and the 1997 DG. _____

_____

3. Amelia S.

Amelia is a 40-year-old woman who fell at home and cut her nose on her coffee table and now presents to the emergency department (ED). She did not lose consciousness but does have a laceration on the bridge of her nose and has had some bleeding through both nostrils. Amelia has a history of hypertension and takes a baby aspirin and hydrochlorothiazide every day. She is allergic to sulfa.

Examination shows an alert, oriented, and pleasant woman; her pulse is 100 and BP is 200/95. She is afebrile. Her neck is supple. She has a 3-cm laceration across the bridge of the nose with blood from the right nostril. There is no blood in the oropharynx. The patient is treated with Steri-Strips and advised that she can take acetaminophen for any pain while the laceration heals.

a. *Identify the chief complaint.* _____

b. *Identify the level of HPI.* _____

c. *Identify the level of ROS.* _____

d. *Identify the level of PFSH.* _____

e. *Identify the level of examination.* _____

f. *Identify the level of MSM.* _____

g. *What is the LOS* using the 1995 DG? _____

4. Jonas W.

Jonas is a 12-year-old white male presenting for an upper right extremity injury, which is not severe. Jonas was last seen a year ago for his annual physical. He fell off his bicycle this afternoon. He has no known drug allergies. His pupils are equal and reactive to light; his arm is not impaired other than minor soft tissue damage. Lungs are clear to auscultation; his abdomen is soft and nontender; there is no hepatosplenomegaly. The physician recommends rest and quiet for the remainder of today. She orders Tylenol for pain and orders the scrapes and bruises to be cleaned and bandaged. No x-ray is needed at this time; the patient's parents will call if necessary.

Code for this E/M service using the 1997 general multisystem examination guidelines. _____

_____

5. Gus B.

Gus, a new patient, is a 55-year-old male who gets intermittent chest pain. The pain is sometimes associated with dyspnea and is usually short-lived. Gus quit smoking 15 years ago, has some alcohol use, and is a draftsman. His mother died at 60 of coronary artery disease. He states he does wheeze at times, but has no GI problems. The physician reviews his patient intake form, and all other systems are negative. Gus is not on any medications.

> **EXAMINATION:** BP: 124/72, pulse: 70, weight: 175, alert, well-developed, neat grooming. Eyes with normal conjunctivae and lids; his extraocular muscles are intact; chest has no rales, wheezes, or rubs; coronary is without murmur, has normal sinus rhythm; abdomen is without masses or tenderness, has normal bowel sounds; good muscle tone in arms and legs. ECG-normal, rate 64; laboratory results show cholesterol is 191.
> **ASSESSMENT:** Palpitations.
> **PLAN:** Holter monitor needed; eliminate caffeine; consider stress test.

Code for this E/M service using the 1995 DG. _____

6. Mitchell H.

Office Note

> **HISTORY:** The patient has not been seen in over a year. He presents with general malaise, fever to 103, and cough occasionally productive of blood-tinged sputum for 4 days. He denies nausea or vomiting. The patient did start a new job recently at an aircraft plant.
> **EXAMINATION:** Temperature, 102.7, weight is 181 lb, BP is 148/84. He is in mild distress. HEENT: Nares are patent. Pharynx is markedly erythematous without exudates or ulcerations. NECK: Supple with anterior cervical lymphadenopathy bilaterally.
> **CHEST:** Examination reveals scattered rhonchi, which clear with cough, no rashes.
> **LABORATORY:** Chest x-ray done here reveals no discrete infiltrates.
> **ASSESSMENT:** 1. Viral syndrome. 2. Acute bronchitis with bronchospasm.
> **PLAN:** Push fluids, suggest Tylenol for fever, antibiotic QID x 10 days. Robitussin DM PRN. Follow-up in 3 days if symptoms do not improve.

Code for this E/M visit using the 1995 DG. _____

7. Arthur M.

Emergency Department

HPI: Arthur, a 16-year-old male, fell and cut his right forearm on a glass door at home. He denies any numbness or weakness of his right upper extremity. He denies any other injury. A dressing was applied at the scene.
PMH: Unremarkable.
PFH: No medical problems that consistently run in the family. Patient is on no medications. No known drug allergies (NKDA).
SH: The patient lives in a safe and reasonable environment. He has no primary care physician. His immunizations are up-to-date per mother.
PE: Wt.: 63 kg; P: 81; R: 18; T: 99; BP: 113/78. Patient is an adolescent male in no acute distress. Hydration is adequate.

Head ☐	Eyes ☐	Ears, nose, throat, mouth ☐	Neck ☐
Respiratory/Chest ☐	CV ☐	Abdomen ☐	Genital/Rectal ☐

MS ☐   Skin ☑ 8 cm laceration into but not penetrating fascial layer.
Neurological ☑ RT UF NVI to M/R/U nerve distribution. 2+ radial pulse.
PROCEDURE: Local anesthetic infiltrated around the wound borders. Wound was irrigated with normal saline. Four subcuticular sutures were placed with 4-0 Vicryl. Wound was then closed with 15 4-0 Prolene for the skin. Tetanus booster was given 0.5 cc IM.

Code for this E/M visit using the 1995 DG. _____

8. Georgia M.

Physician Office

HISTORY: The patient was referred by her primary care provider for evaluation of a lesion of the right scalp and left eyelid. The patient also was concerned about a lesion of her right neck. She is a new patient to this office.
PMH: The patient is healthy with no chronic illnesses aside from high cholesterol. She is peri-menopausal. The patient takes multivitamins and Zocor.
SH: She is a manager for a beach resort and spends a great deal of time outdoors. She states she wears cosmetics and moisturizer with SPF 15. She applies sunscreen to her arms and legs if she is out for prolonged periods of time. She denies smoking and drinks three to five drinks per week.
PE: The lesion of the right scalp appeared consistent with hemangioma with an adjacent lesion suggestive of a sebaceous nevus. Scalp lesions measured 0.4 cm by 0.4 cm. Patient also has a 0.3-cm lesion of the right neck and a 1-mm lesion of the left eyelid. The neck is supple with no lymphadenopathy; her eyes are equal, round, and reactive to light; and her head shows no other anomalies.
PLAN: I plan to biopsy the lesions. The patient is to follow up after pathology results are obtained.

Code for this E/M visit using the 1995 DG. _____

9. Issiah S.

Established Patient

> **HPI:** The patient has not been seen for over 2 years and is here today because of warts on the left heel and right third toe. He has trimmed these at home and tried over-the-counter wart treatments without success. He states that these are irritated when wearing shoes and cause pain and bleeding at times. He has seen his family physician and had these removed, but they keep returning and increasing in size. He wants these removed.
>
> **ROS:** Patient is well developed and in no acute distress. Patient does not complain of any other skin abnormalities. He has no allergies and has not been sick within the last 3 months. He takes no medication other than a baby aspirin and multivitamins.
>
> **PE:** One 0.5-cm wart is located on the left heel and another 0.3-cm wart is on the right third toe.
>
> **PLAN:** Laser ablation. Patient to follow up in 10 days.

Code for this E/M visit using the 1995 DG. _____

10. Roger E.

Established Patient

> Roger had a coronary artery bypass graft 6 months ago. I have seen this patient each year for his annual physical. He is 60 years old and did well following the surgery but is here today because of a 2-day history of stomach pain. He is feeling weak and tired. He does not have indigestion or heartburn. He has no known allergies. The patient takes furosemide, potassium, and losartan. He does not have chest pain or shortness of breath.
>
> **EXAMINATION:** BP is 140/80, heart rate is 78, weight is 170.
>
> **EYES:** PERRLA.
>
> **LUNGS:** Clear to auscultation.
>
> **HEART:** Without murmur.
>
> **GI:** Soft, no organomegaly.
>
> Blood work done today is normal. Patient will require additional testing to determine the cause of his pain.

Code for this E/M visit using the 1995 DG. _____

INTERNET RESEARCH

1. Find Medicare's Internet-based training module for fraud and abuse. First go to www.cms.gov. Click on the "Outreach and Education" box all the way to the left. In the search box in the right-hand corner, type in "Internet based training for fraud and abuse." Below you will see Medicare learning network for fraud and abuse.
2. Find CMS quarterly provider updates by first going to www.cms.hhs.gov/quarterlyproviderupdates, then reviewing the list of updates by date on the left.
3. Go to www.cms.gov and in the search box type "avoiding Medicare fraud and abuse." It will bring up a Medicare learning network article about fraud and abuse issues for physicians.

MEDICAL CODING LAB Remember to use the coding activities at **Medicalcodinglab.com** for extra practice on what you have just learned and to test your knowledge.

CHAPTER 15

CPT: Anesthesia Codes

Anesthesia services can be some of the most difficult services to code, especially from a billing perspective. Coding for anesthesia services is not routinely done by physician practices or health information management (HIM) coders; it is considered a coding specialty. However, it is important for all medical coders to have a basic understanding of this important topic.

The administration of anesthesia causes the patient to lose the ability to feel pain. The administered drug or other medical intervention causes partial or complete loss of sensation, with or without loss of consciousness. In CPT, anesthesia codes are grouped anatomically by body area, first in the order of the head down to the feet, and then from the shoulder to the hand.

Chapter 15 in *Conquer Medical Coding* explains the assignment of CPT anesthesia codes with appropriate HCPCS modifiers and physical status modifiers based on anesthesia procedural statements. The chapter also covers the following information:

- The organization, guidelines, and key modifiers for the Anesthesia section in CPT
- The various anesthesia techniques: general, local, nerve block, regional, conscious sedation, and monitored anesthesia care (MAC)
- The concept of a complete anesthesia service
- The common coding mistakes and missed billing opportunities when reporting anesthesia services
- When anesthesia modifiers and qualifying circumstances are reported and the documentation necessary to code anesthesia services
- How to calculate anesthesia time units and fees based on prescribed formulas

CODE IT!

Assign all pertinent procedure codes and modifiers.

1. _____ Biopsy of the clavicle under general anesthesia

2. _____ Cesarean section of a 25-year-old who had no epidural during labor, performed by certified registered nurse anesthetist (CRNA)

3. _____ Anesthesia provided by anesthesiologist for arthroscopic meniscus repair of the right knee

4. _____ Transurethral resection of the prostate

5. _____ Repair of cleft palate under general anesthesia

6. _____ Nasal septoplasty for deviated septum

7. _____ Total left knee replacement surgery

8. _____ Anesthesia provided by anesthesiologist for dressing change of the lower leg

9. _____ Orchiopexy in a 3-year-old boy

10. _____ Vasectomy in a 35-year-old man

MULTIPLE CHOICE

Select the option that best provides the correct code, completes the statement, or answers the question.

1. When does anesthesia time begin?
   A. When the anesthesiologist meets with the patient preoperatively
   B. When the anesthesiologist has the patient fully anesthetized
   C. When the anesthesiologist begins to prepare the patient for the induction of anesthesia
   D. When the anesthesiologist begins to prepare the patient for coming out of anesthesia

2. Open procedure is performed to revise a total hip arthroplasty on a patient with uncontrolled diabetes and long-term congestive heart failure. The patient is 78 years old. What is the correct coding to use for this situation?
   A. 01214–P2
   B. 01215–P3, +99100
   C. 01214–P3
   D. 01214–P3, +99100

3. After several weeks of upper abdominal pain, a patient has surgery for a cholecystectomy. The patient has type 2, controlled diabetes. What is the correct coding to use for this situation?
   A. 00790–P2
   B. 00731
   C. 00731–P2
   D. 00750–P2

4. Because the patient spent many hours of labor without any medication for pain, and because the baby was not moving into the birth canal adequately for a vaginal delivery, the decision was made to perform a cesarean section under general anesthesia. What is the correct coding to use for this situation?
   A. 01961
   B. 01961, +01968
   C. +01968
   D. 01967, +01968

5. If a CRNA performs MAC during a breast biopsy under the medical direction of an anesthesiologist, report the CRNA's services as:
   A. 00454 QX, QS
   B. 00400 QX
   C. 00402 QS
   D. 00400 QX, QS

6. The anesthesiologist personally performs MAC during insertion of an implantable central venous access (CVA) device. What is the correct coding to use for this situation?
   A. 00532 AA, QS
   B. 00530 AA, QS
   C. 00532, +99140
   D. 00530, +99140

7. The anesthesiologist performs MAC for bronchoscopy with biopsy on a patient with a history of congestive heart failure. What is the correct coding to use for this situation?
   A. 00522, AA, G9
   B. 00520, AA, G9
   C. 00522, AA, G8
   D. 00520, AA, G8

8. The patient is 55 years old with a diagnosis of a 5.5-cm aortoiliac aneurysm. She underwent general anesthesia for the endovascular repair of the aneurysm with pump oxygenator. What is the correct coding to use for this situation?
   A. 00560
   B. 00561
   C. 00562
   D. 00563

9. Radical inguinal orchiectomy of the left testicle occurs with insertion of prosthesis for a 73-year-old male with hypertension and prostate cancer metastatic to the left testicle under general anesthesia. What is the correct coding to use for this situation?
   A. 00910
   B. 00920
   C. 00914
   D. 00922

10. Which three services are not included in the anesthesia code and can be billed separately?
   A. Swan-Ganz, postoperative visits, ECG
   B. Blood pressure, intra-arterial monitoring, Swan-Ganz
   C. Oximetry, capnography, mass spectrometry
   D. Intra-arterial monitoring, central venous monitoring, Swan-Ganz

SHORT ANSWER

Answer the following questions.

1. Name one service other than administering anesthesia that is included in anesthesia codes.

   _____

   _____

2. A patient with advanced carcinoma of the esophagus with widespread metastases has general anesthesia for a partial esophagectomy. Code for the anesthesia and any relevant modifier(s). _____

   _____

3. A well-conditioned 22-year-old athlete has anesthesia administered for extensive debridement of the shoulder joint by arthroscopy. Which code is used? _____

   _____

4. List two modifiers (not physical status modifiers or qualifying circumstances) that describe anesthesia services. _____

_____

5. Situations that significantly affect the character of an anesthesia service are represented by codes referred to as: _____

_____

6. The anesthesiologist met preoperatively with the patient to discuss the anesthesia services and to discuss the patient's condition. How would these preoperative services be reported?

_____

7. The physical status modifier was appended to both the anesthesia code and the surgery code. Is this correct? Why or why not? _____

_____

8. What is the anesthesia code for coronary artery bypass graft with pump oxygenator? _____

_____

9. What is the anesthesia code for a diagnostic arthroscopy of the knee? _____

_____

10. After receiving neuraxial labor anesthesia, the patient underwent a cesarean delivery. The coder reported only code 01968. Is the coder correct? _____

_____

CASE STUDIES

1. Joanna A.

> **ANESTHESIA:** General with mask.
> **ANESTHESIOLOGIST:** William B., MD.
> **COMPLICATIONS:** None.
> **PREOPERATIVE and POSTOPERATIVE DIAGNOSIS:** Mild dysplasia with positive high-risk human papillomavirus (HPV).
> **OPERATION:** Loop electrosurgical excision procedure (LEEP).
> **PROCEDURE:** After adequate general anesthesia, the patient was placed in the dorsal lithotomy position, using candy cane stirrups. I put the speculum in and cleaned the cervix with vinegar. She had a small amount of central white epithelium. I injected the cervix with 4 cc of lidocaine with epinephrine and took the small, 1-cm loop and made one central pass, which removed the transformation zone to a depth of 1 cm. I then cauterized the cone bed and applied Monsel solution. The procedure was terminated at this point. The plastic, coated speculum that had been placed at the beginning was removed.

Code for the anesthesia service. _____

2. Maryann D.

> **ANESTHESIA:** General.
> **ANESTHETIST:** Marsha N., CRNA.
> **PROCEDURE:** Below the knee amputation, right leg.
> **FINDINGS AND INDICATIONS:** Maryann D., a 41-year-old white female, had a large right leg laceration that became infected and is now gangrenous because of lack of medical care for the injury. She now requires a below-the-knee amputation under general anesthesia to save the leg.

Code for the anesthesia service. _____

3. Anna P.

> **ANESTHESIA:** MAC and local anesthetic.
> **ANESTHETIST:** Leslie L., CRNA.
> **ANESTHESIOLOGIST:** Sean Black, MD.
> **PREOPERATIVE and POSTOPERATIVE DIAGNOSIS:** Visual field impairment, Blepharochalasis upper lid.
> **OPERATION:** Upper lid blepharoplasty.
> **PROCEDURE:** With the patient under suitable IV sedation, in the supine position on the operating table, a pattern with French curl was drawn on the patient's eyelids with lateral to medial distances from the lid–lash margin of 4 mm and 8 mm in the central portion on each side. Thereafter, local anesthetic was injected—a 50/50 solution of 1% Xylocaine plus 0.25% Marcaine, 1:200,000 epinephrine. The patient was prepped with Shur-Clens solution and draped aseptically. Thereafter, excision of the excess skin on the right upper eyelid and left upper eyelid were undertaken. Removal of the medial and lateral fat pads of the upper lids was undertaken with cauterization of all vessels and bases of fat pads. The patient's vision was not affected by this during the operation except to improve the visual fields from drooping lids. Repair was undertaken with 6-0 nylon. The patient tolerated the procedure well.

Code for the CRNA. _____

4. Herschel M.

> **ANESTHESIA:** General Buck, MD.
> **PREOPERATIVE DIAGNOSIS:** Left lung lesion.
> Herschel M., a mentally unstable patient, requires a bronchoscopy to determine if a lesion on the left lung is malignant or benign. Bronchoscopy procedures are commonly done under local anesthetic, but because of the patient's mental condition general anesthesia will be provided.

What modifier will best represent this scenario? Keep in mind that a carrier will most likely deny a general anesthesia code billed with a bronchoscopy code. _____

5. Anouk M.

> **ANESTHESIA:** General.
> **ANESTHESIOLOGIST:** George H., MD.
> **PREOPERATIVE DIAGNOSIS:** Appendicitis.
> An emergency appendectomy is performed on a 75-year-old patient with insulin-dependent diabetes that is not under control. The anesthesiologist begins administration of the general anesthesia at 10:00 a.m. and completes the anesthesia services at 10:45 a.m.

List the key elements. Indicate "none" if not applicable.

a. Anesthesia procedure code: _____

b. Physical status modifier: _____

c. Qualifying circumstances code: _____

d. Anesthesia modifier(s): _____

e. Calculate time units (15-minute increments): _____

6. Charles M.

> **ANESTHESIA:** General.
> **ANESTHESIOLOGIST:** Karen M., MD.
> **PREOPERATIVE DIAGNOSIS:** Dental caries
> Charles M., a 3-year-old child, has developed significant and progressive destructive disease of his teeth because of decay caused by the use of a bottled formula. He now requires that his dental caries be filled and caps placed. He will be placed under general anesthesia provided by an anesthesiologist.

Code for the anesthesia service. _____

7. Harrison A.

> **ANESTHESIA:** General.
> **ANESTHESIOLOGIST:** Karen M., MD.
> **ANESTHETIST:** Archer Stabile, CRNA.
> **PREOPERATIVE DIAGNOSIS:** Left bundle branch block.
> Harrison, a 70-year-old patient with senile dementia, is in the hospital for insertion of a permanent dual-chamber pacemaker. Mr. A. is very combative and will not allow anyone to treat him. After a lengthy discussion with his cardiologist, Mr. A. is calm and agrees to go to the operating room where the decision is made to use general anesthesia versus moderate sedation or local anesthetic. The CRNA provides the anesthesia under the direction of the anesthesiologist.

Code for both the anesthesiologist and the CRNA. _____

8. Jacob S.

> **PREOPERATIVE DIAGNOSIS:** Right chronic otitis media.
> **PROCEDURE:** Right tympanomastoidectomy.
> **ANESTHESIOLOGIST:** Ralph O., MD.
> **INDICATIONS:** Jacob, an 80-year-old patient, has a history of aortic valve replacement and congestive heart failure, diabetes, and hypertension. The patient was brought to the operating room, identified, and placed on the table in the supine position. General anesthesia was induced.

Code for the anesthesia service. _____

9. Frieda M.

> **PREOPERATIVE DIAGNOSIS:** Mass, upper outer left breast.
> **PROCEDURE:** Excision of left breast mass.
> **ANESTHETIST:** Tanesha H, CRNA.
> **INDICATIONS:** Frieda M. is a 55-year-old woman who discovered a lump on her breast several
> months ago. She is here now for removal of the mass in her breast. After intravenous adminis-
> tration of general anesthesia, a 2.5-cm skin incision was made and a flap raised between sub-
> cutaneous fibrofatty tissue and breast tissue until the mass was identified.

Code for the anesthesia service. _____

10. Peter R.

> **PREOPERATIVE DIAGNOSIS:** Chordee.
> **PROCEDURE:** Repair of chordee.
> **INDICATIONS:** Peter is a 14-month-old boy with congenital chordee. He was brought to the op-
> erating room, identified, prepped, and draped in the usual sterile manner and placed in the
> supine position under general anesthesia. The examination of the penis under anesthesia re-
> vealed a 90-degree chordee with a ventral bend.

Code for the anesthesia service. _____

INTERNET RESEARCH

1. The AAPC certifies medical coders in various medical specialties. Visit www.aapc.com
   and list the surgery-related specialty coding certifications that are available. What are the
   requirements to become anesthesia certified?
2. Visit the Anesthesia Resources website at www.anesres.com. Search for the key phrase "OIG."
   What is the issue that the OIG is warning surgeons and anesthesiologists about?
3. Visit the ASA website (www.asahq.org. Under "Quality & Practice Management," select
   "Standards & Guidelines" and then "Anesthesia Care," and then the pdf "Basic Anesthesia
   Monitoring." In Section 3, Ventilation, find how ventilation is evaluated in regional or local
   anesthesia.
4. Visit the Anesthesia Resources website at www.anesres.com/reports. Select the link "Getting
   Paid for Post-op Pain Blocks." When does the payer First Coast allow separate reimbursement
   for nerve blocks? Name three documentation strategies explained in the article.

MEDICAL CODING LAB Remember to use the coding activities at **Medicalcodinglab.com** for extra practice
on what you have just learned and to test your knowledge.

CPT: Surgery Codes

Chapter 16 in *Conquer Medical Coding* lays the groundwork for the surgical chapters that follow in the text by discussing surgical concepts, terminology, and guidelines that are applied to all surgical coding, regardless of surgical specialty. Codes located in the surgery section of CPT include invasive diagnostic or therapeutic procedures performed in a physician office, clinic, surgery center, or hospital. Each surgical section is subdivided by body areas, working from the head to the feet and then further subdivided by type of procedure. In addition to explaining these topics, Chapter 16 explains the following:

- The components of a surgical package
- The distinction between the CPT and Medicare definitions of surgical package
- The therapeutic versus diagnostic procedures and when to assign codes
- The definition and examples of "separate procedure"
- How to identify whether a procedure is incidental or separately reported
- How to use the available references to correctly report surgical services and modifiers
- The difference between modifiers for physician use and hospital outpatient use
- How to correctly assign modifiers for services performed during the global period
- How to correctly assign CPT codes to basic procedural statements

CODE IT!

Supply the correct codes for the following.

1. _____ Removal of foreign body from the nose

2. _____ Patch closure of ventricular septal defect

3. _____ Removal of foreign body from external auditory canal, general anesthesia

4. _____ Mastoidectomy, modified radical, right ear

5. _____ Bone marrow biopsy

6. _____ Tympanoplasty, right ear

7. _____ Repair of ruptured spleen

8. _____ Cochlear implant

9. _____ Vasovasorrhaphy

10. _____ Surgical treatment of first trimester missed abortion

MULTIPLE CHOICE

Select the option that best provides the correct code, completes the statement, or answers the question.

1. Partial colectomy is provided to a patient whose tumor adheres to the blood vessels. An additional 60 minutes was required over the normal operative time to remove the tumor. The surgeon documented the circumstances that required the additional time. What modifier should be appended to the surgery code?
   A. −58
   B. −22
   C. −62
   D. −78

2. The partial colectomy patient is now seeing his surgeon in the office 1 month after the surgery because he is short of breath and is sure that it is related to the surgery. The surgeon examines the patient and determines that the patient's issue is not related to the surgery. How should the surgeon report this service?
   A. The surgeon cannot report an E/M code because of the global period.
   B. The surgeon uses the E/M code with modifier −59.
   C. The surgeon uses the E/M code with modifier −24.
   D. The surgeon uses the surgery code with modifier −55.

3. In CPT, the code description that follows the semicolon is:
   A. Not part of the parent code
   B. Included in the description of the indented code(s)
   C. Not included in the description of the indented code(s)
   D. Incidental

4. The indication portion (preoperative diagnosis) listed on the operative report is used to describe:
   A. The surgical procedure
   B. The medical necessity for the procedure
   C. The patient's status intraoperatively
   D. The severity of the procedure being performed

5. When a patient is in a postoperative period and returns to the operating room for an unrelated procedure by the same physician, which modifier would be used?
   A. −59
   B. −79
   C. −78
   D. −62

6. Which of the following modifiers would be used with an E/M encounter when the physician determines that the patient will need major surgery on the next day?
   A. −25
   B. −24
   C. −57
   D. −58

7. A 12-year-old is seen by his family doctor for a laceration on his arm. The doctor did a layered closure of the arm (12034). The patient also mentioned he has begun to develop acne; he is very self-conscious and has an odd rash on his leg. The doctor provided an E/M service and reported a wound repair code. How will the doctor report his services?
   A. E/M code with modifier –25
   B. E/M code, wound repair code
   C. Wound repair code
   D. E/M code with modifier –25 and wound repair code

8. Designated separate procedure means:
   A. You cannot report the procedure if it is the only procedure performed.
   B. You can report the procedure if it is the only procedure performed or if it is performed in a separate site or during a separate session from another more major procedure.
   C. You can always report it separately.
   D. You can report it separately if you report it on a separate line in the claim form.

9. Which of the following are used to assist in determining the physician's best course of treatment?
   A. Diagnostic procedures
   B. Therapeutic procedures
   C. Operative report
   D. Surgery modifier

10. Modifier –47 is reported by the:
    A. Surgeon with the surgery code
    B. Surgeon with the anesthesia code
    C. Anesthesiologist with the surgery code
    D. Anesthesiologist with the anesthesia code

SHORT ANSWER

Answer the following questions.

1. A 40-year-old woman fell at home and cut her nose on her coffee table, causing a laceration on the bridge of her nose. What code range will be used to report a simple repair of the laceration?

   _____

   _____

2. An accidental fall from a bike caused the 10-year-old patient to require repair of the tympanic membrane. What is the code for the repair? _____

3. A 73-year-old woman was seen 4 years ago by her endocrinologist for diabetes and has returned to see her endocrinologist again. Is she a new or established patient? _____

   _____

4. A 40-year-old woman has had vaginal bleeding for over 4 weeks. After evaluation by her gynecologist, she undergoes a diagnostic hysteroscopy. What is the code for the procedure? _____

   _____

5. An 80-year-old man who has had osteoarthritis for over 30 years undergoes a total knee replacement. What is the code for the knee replacement? _____

   _____

6. A dermatologist provides a destruction procedure of a premalignant lesion of the back. What is the code for the procedure? _____

_____

7. A fall caused an injury to the patient's neck. An x-ray revealed damage to the jugular vein of the neck. An open (direct) repair of a neck vein is performed. What is the code for the procedure? _____

8. After an evaluation of a lesion, the physician performs an excision of a 4.0-cm malignant lesion of the chest. What is the code for the excision? _____

_____

9. A 40-year-old female patient has suffered from having overly large breasts, which have caused back pain and skin abrasions on her shoulders. She is here today to have a reduction mammaplasty. What is the code for the procedure? _____

10. After years of incontinence, the patient is having a cystourethroscopy procedure with biopsy of the bladder. What is the code for the procedure? _____

_____

CASE STUDIES

1. Tyesha J.

   Tyesha, a neonate, was born at 36 weeks' gestation. The child was in noticeable physical distress and was taken to the NICU for monitoring and tests. The physician reported the service with code 99468, which is correct.

   The physician also wanted to report the modifier 52 with that code. Is she correct? _____

   _____

2. Roberta S.

   > **PREOPERATIVE DIAGNOSIS:** Mammographic abnormality of the left and right breast.
   > **PROCEDURE:** Needle-localized left excisional breast biopsy to left and right breast.
   > **OPERATION:** After adequate sedation was achieved, the patient's left breast was prepped with Betadine and draped in a sterile fashion. A curvilinear incision, just inferior to the localizing needle, was made with a knife. Dissection was carried down bluntly. An Allis clamp was then placed on the specimen and sharp dissection carried around the perimeter, providing a generous core of tissue, surrounding the top of the localizing needle. The identical services were provided on the right breast.

   What modifier will be appended to the breast biopsy code? _____

3. Marvin H.

   Marvin was brought back to the operating room during the postoperative period by the same physician to repair a percutaneous gastrostomy tube inserted 4 days ago. The surgeon used a transabdominal approach to suture a leak that had developed in the area of the tube.

   What modifier should the surgeon append to the surgery code? _____

4. Adriana O.

> **PREOPERATIVE DIAGNOSIS:** Fractured patella.
> **PROCEDURE:** Repair of patellar fracture.
> While shoveling snow at her neighbor's home, Adriana fell onto her right knee and experienced great pain. An x-ray revealed a fracture of the patella. With Adriana under general anesthesia, an incision was made, revealing the patella, which was severely fragmented. The patella was wired and the surrounding tissue was repaired and irrigated.

Identify the sentence that determines whether this procedure was performed as an open or closed repair. _____

_____

5. George R.

George was stabbed in the chest and went to the emergency department (ED) of the hospital. The surgeon removes the knife and explores the wound to determine the extent of the penetration. He finds that the knife penetrated the pleura and a thoracotomy is necessary to further explore the chest area.

Will the surgeon report wound repair or thoracotomy? _____

_____

6. Ellen M.

> **PREOPERATIVE DIAGNOSIS:** Atelectasis of the right lower lobe.
> **PROCEDURE:** Diagnostic flexible bronchoscopy with endobronchial ultrasound.
> Ellen is a 50-year-old woman who has suffered a loss of air in the right lower lobe of the lung. The bronchoscope was passed through the endotracheal tube down to the carina and the ultrasound transducer was passed through a channel of the bronchoscope. Some swollen tissue was seen in the right lower lobe and cell washings were done.

The physician reported codes 31622 and +31620. Can modifier 51 be reported with the secondary code? _____

7. Henry E.

Henry, a 74-year-old patient, was referred to a cardiologist for a consultation by his family doctor. The family doctor is asking for the cardiologist's opinion on the patient's condition. Henry's symptoms were chest pain and left arm pain. He has had chest pain for several months but insists that is because of his many years of eating chili peppers and that it is a gastrointestinal problem. Once the added problem of left arm pain became an issue, he agreed to see the cardiologist. Based on the cardiologist's examination and testing, Henry was admitted to the hospital for further tests. The cardiologist wants to report the consultation code with modifier 57.

Is the cardiologist correct? _____

8. Caroline M.

Caroline, a 40-year-old patient, presented to the physician's office with a chief complaint of abdominal pain for over 6 months. The initial examination indicated a possible mass and an exploratory laparotomy was scheduled. During the exploratory laparotomy the physician discovered a 3.5-cm tumor, which was excised.

The surgeon wants to report the exploratory laparotomy code 49000 (separate procedure) and 49203 excision of intra-abdominal tumor. Is the surgeon correct? _____

9. Andrew S.

Andrew was seriously wounded in a bar fight and was subsequently seen in the ED. He was stabbed on the right side of the chest. The physician in the ED needs to make an incision into the thoracic cavity to determine if there is greater damage from the knife wound than what appears from just the wound exploration.

Should the coder report a thoracotomy code or a thoracostomy code? _____

_____

10. Leah T.

> **PREOPERATIVE DIAGNOSIS:** Left rotator cuff tear.
> **OPERATION:** Left shoulder arthroscopy, repair rotator cuff, subacromial decompression.
> **PROCEDURE:** The patient was placed in a beach chair with 10 lb. of distraction. Three portals were created anteriorly, laterally, and posteriorly, and the 3M pump was utilized.
> The glenohumeral joint revealed that there was at least a tear to the supraspinatus and infraspinatus measuring 6 cm. The articular surfaces were normal. Attention was then in the subacromial space as a bursectomy ensued with a wand and shaver. The C-A ligament was incised from the anterior acromion as the acromion was found to have spurs. It was then converted to a type I and flat acromion with a burr. A fragment of the C-A was excised. The supraspinatus was then found to have a 6-cm stellate-type multiple planar tear off the greater tuberosity, which was prepared with a burr to bleeding bone. The rotator cuff was repaired anatomically after doing an extended portal: first side-to-side with fiberwire #2 back to the tuberosity using three Spiral Locs anchors and #2 Orthocord and Krakow sutures. All knots were very secure and stable with completion as the shoulder was taken through the range of motion.

Was this procedure performed as an open or endoscopic procedure and which shoulder was treated? What type of sutures were used? _____

_____

_____

INTERNET RESEARCH

1. Go to the following website and determine what the global surgery days are for procedure code 31255: www.cms.gov/Medicare/Medicare-Fee-for-Service-Payment/PhysicianFeeSched/index.html and select PFS-Relative-Value-Files.
2. Modifier −59 is scrutinized by Medicare and is often found to be abused. Read the following excerpt from the Medicare Carrier Manual for a detailed description and examples of proper use: www.cms.hhs.gov/NationalCorrectCodInitEd/Downloads/modifier59.pdf
3. Locate the National Correct Coding Initiative Policy Manual on the CMS website and read Chapter 1, "General Correct Coding Policies for National Correct Coding Initiative Policy Manual for Medicare Services." This chapter is an easy read and reinforces what was discussed in this chapter along with explanation of commonly used modifiers.

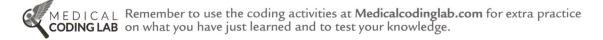 MEDICAL CODING LAB — Remember to use the coding activities at **Medicalcodinglab.com** for extra practice on what you have just learned and to test your knowledge.

CPT: Integumentary System

Chapter 17 in *Conquer Medical Coding* focuses on the procedural coding and terminology of surgical cases involving procedures performed on the skin and subcutaneous tissue as well as the breasts and nails. Chapter 17 also explains the following:

- The steps in assigning procedure codes for the surgical procedures common to the integumentary system: incision and drainage, biopsy, destruction, debridement, excision, repair, and Mohs micrographic surgery
- The guidelines for coding excision of lesions
- The difference among simple, intermediate, and complex wound repairs
- How to accurately calculate measurements for lesion excisions
- The four types of debridement codes
- The difference between selective, nonselective, and surgical wound debridement

CODE IT!

Assign all pertinent procedure codes, modifiers, and HCPCS codes.

1. _____ Breast lumpectomy of a malignant tumor.

2. _____ Excision of a 2.6-cm benign lesion on the patient's chin.

3. _____ Removal of a 1.2-cm mole from the neck by shave technique.

4. _____ Injection of eight scars of the neck, ear, face, and chest. The patient is 1 year status post four-wheeler accident where the patient struck tree branches.

5. _____ Repair of a disrupted surgical incision site with simple repair and Steri-Strips.

6. _____ A Mohs micrographic surgery of a lesion on the arm, first stage, four tissue blocks.

7. _____ Laser destruction of a premalignant 1.5-cm lesion of the shoulder and 0.5-cm lesion of the back of the neck.

8. _____ An 84-year-old nursing home patient bumped into the corner of a coffee table, sustaining a superficial wound. Three weeks later, the wound appeared to be healing but she scraped off the scab, causing granulation tissue to form. The physician performed a chemical cauterization of granulation tissue using silver nitrate on the left lower leg.

9. _____ A 37-year-old male presents to the primary care physician office requesting removal of his skin tags. These have been present for many years and are growing in number. Many of them are interfering with daily activities such as shaving and are rubbing on clothing. Skin tags are located on the neck, face, axillae, forearms, and groin. Ten tags were removed sharply by scalpel from the face and neck, and 18 tags were electrocauterized from the axillae, forearms, and groin.

10. _____ The patient has a large nonhealing radiation ulcer of the left chest. After excision, a defect remains that is repaired with a pedicled latissimus muscle flap. Code for the muscle flap.

MULTIPLE CHOICE

Select the option that best provides the correct code, completes the statement, or answers the question.

1. One benign lesion measuring 0.5 cm is removed from the arm and another benign lesion measuring 0.8 cm is removed from the hand. What is the correct way to code this situation?
   A. 11401, 11400–51
   B. 11421, 11400–51
   C. 11402
   D. 11421, 11420–51

2. Intermediate repair to the left elbow wound—3 cm. Debridement—left leg wound, including bone, 20 sq. cm. What is the correct way to code this situation?
   A. 11001
   B. 11043
   C. 12032, 11044
   D. 11012

3. A boy was shaving and cut his neck—1.5-cm laceration. Bleeding came from the skin edges. No muscle was exposed. The laceration was sutured in one layer. What is the correct way to code this situation?
   A. 12001
   B. 12041
   C. 12011
   D. 12002

4. Complex repair of a 10-cm laceration—forehead, 6-cm laceration—right cheek, 5-cm laceration—chin, 9-cm laceration—dorsum, right hand. What is the correct way to code this situation?
   A. 13132, 13133; 13132; 13132, 13133
   B. 12056
   C. 2054; 12053; 12052; 12044
   D. 13132, 13133x5

5. The patient arrived with a 6-cm wound on his left arm, requiring layered closure and extensive undermining of tissue in all directions. What is the correct way to code this situation?
   A. 13121
   B. 12032
   C. 12031
   D. 13101

6. Excision of a 70 sq. cm burn scar on the arm and elbow, with preparation of the recipient site. A split-thickness graft, 100 sq. cm, is used to cover the defect. What is the correct way to code this situation?
   A. 14300, 15100
   B. 15100, 15101
   C. 15002, 15100
   D. 14300

7. The patient's nostril was retracted because of a scar. The scar was excised and the dorsal nasal flap was used to repair a 2 sq. cm defect caused by the excision. What is the correct way to code this situation?
   A. 15260
   B. 14040, 15120
   C. 14060, 15120
   D. 14060

8. In the previous example, suppose a 4 sq. cm. full-thickness skin graft was required to close the donor site of the flap. What code is used for the skin graft only?
   A. 15240
   B. 15260
   C. 15120
   D. 15004

9. A patient with basal cell carcinoma on her neck requires eradication of the 1.9-cm tumor. The first stage excision was divided into four blocks. Upon microscopic review by the surgeon, a tumor remained in three of the four blocks. A second stage was excised containing the residual tumor. This was divided into three blocks and the surgeon again provided the pathology microscopic examination. What is the correct way to code this situation?
   A. 17313, +17314–51
   B. 17311, +17312–51
   C. 17313, +17314
   D. 17311, +17312

10. What code range is used to code for exploration of penetrating trauma without laparotomy or thoracotomy?
    A. 12002–13153
    B. 20100–20103
    C. 32095–32160
    D. 49000–49010

SHORT ANSWER

Answer the following questions.

1. A patient has a skin lesion on the right forearm. The lesion will be excised and biopsied. Can you report both the excision and the biopsy? _____

    _____

2. Code for the intermediate repair of a 4-cm laceration on the right leg and a 3-cm laceration on the trunk. _____

3. The patient underwent partial mastectomy 2 weeks ago for a malignant tumor. She presents today for placement of a radiotherapy afterloading expandable balloon catheter. What is the correct code for this procedure? _____

_____

4. A W-plasty represents what type of repair? _____

_____

5. After falling off a motorcycle, the patient required a 130 sq. cm. split-thickness skin graft to his trunk. What is the correct code(s) for this procedure? _____

_____

6. A patient with a necrotizing soft tissue infection on his abdominal wall requires debridement without fascial closure. What is the correct code for this procedure? _____

_____

7. Code for the destruction of 10 premalignant lesions via cryosurgery. _____

_____

8. Code for the destruction of 17 premalignant lesions via cryosurgery. _____

_____

9. Code for MOHS surgery performed on the patient's head, which was accomplished in one stage utilizing six blocks. _____

_____

10. A patient underwent breast reconstruction with TRAM and supercharging. Do you need one or two codes to code for this procedure correctly? _____

_____

CASE STUDIES

1. Tanya T.

> **PREOPERATIVE DIAGNOSIS:** Breast hypertrophy.
> **PROCEDURE PERFORMED:** Bilateral reduction mammoplasty.
> **HISTORY:** This 22-year-old white female, who is otherwise healthy, has been bothered by the weight and length of her breasts. She has been counseled on several occasions regarding her options. Because Tanya is very unhappy with the size, shape, and appearance of her breasts, she has requested a breast lift with a modest reduction of the breast volume.
> **DESCRIPTION OF PROCEDURE:** Once adequate general and local anesthesia and vasoconstriction were obtained, the incisions were then scoured with a #15C blade. A 52-mm circular cookie cutter was used to mark the impression of the new nipple–areola, which was then scoured. The inferior pedicle, which was marked 8 cm in width centered over the breast meridian, was then sharply de-epithelialized. The right breast was approached first and an

identical procedure was performed bilaterally, so only one will be dictated. Once the inferior pedicle had been de-epithelialized, the parenchymal resection was then begun, dividing the full thickness of skin. The superior breast skin flap was then elevated at the level of the breast capsule and dissected toward the clavicle, leaving a very wide base to the central inferior pedicle. Sequential debulking of the inferomedial and inferolateral breast quadrants was then done, and the excess breast tissue was weighed sequentially. A portion of the central upper breast tissue was then reduced. The breast specimen was then combined and the weight totaled. There were no palpable or visible parenchymal abnormalities. Hemostasis was obtained with Bovie electrocautery. There was excellent hemostasis on both sides. The breast wound was then irrigated with copious amounts of bacitracin antibiotic irrigation and rinsed. Hemostasis was again rechecked. PDS layered closure was then effected with interrupted deep dermal sutures of 3-0 Monocryl followed by interrupted dermal sutures of 4-0 Monocryl and running subcuticular suture of 4-0 Monocryl in the inframammary crease closure. The new nipple site was marked at approximately 22 cm in the breast meridian from the sternal notch.

A 40-cm diameter circular impression was made and the central core fat and skin were removed with a #15 blade and sent with each specimen to pathology in formalin. The nipple–areola was then brought out, secured to the skin with interrupted deep dermal sutures 4-0 Monocryl, followed by running cuticular suture of 5-0 Monocryl. The skin flaps and nipple–areola appeared to be well perfused. Incisions were then dressed with Mastisol and flesh-toned Steri-Strips.

Identify the physician CPT codes. _____

2. Ahmed A.

PREOPERATIVE DIAGNOSIS: Traumatic scars, right face, 2 cm.
PROCEDURES: Complex wound revision 2 cm.
OPERATION: The patient was taken to the OR and placed in the supine position. The patient was prepped and draped. The 2-cm scar was then excised in elliptical fashion and closed in layers using 5-0 Monocryl and 6-0 nylon mattress sutures. Steri-Strips were applied to the two wound revisions.

Identify the physician CPT codes. _____

3. Hachiro C.

PREOPERATIVE DIAGNOSIS: Nevus sebaceous, right scalp.
PROCEDURE: Excision of nevus, right scalp, 2 cm. Complex wound closure, 6 cm.
OPERATION: The patient was previously marked in the preoperative area. He was prepped and draped. The lesion was excised elliptically and brought together. It was apparent that the defect would be closed under a fair amount of tension. Wide undermining was performed both bluntly and sharply using cautery. Galeal scoring was performed as well. During the scoring process, the bleeder was divided at the superior aspect. This was cauterized. The defect was closed in layers using 2-0 Monocryl and 4-0 Prolene. The patient was awakened and taken to recovery.

Identify the physician CPT codes. _____

4. Marta S.

PREOPERATIVE DIAGNOSIS: Abscess of breast.
PROCEDURE: Exploration of left breast with drainage of deep abscess.
OPERATION: General anesthesia was administered and the patient's left breast was prepped and draped in the usual sterile fashion. The previous incision lines were reopened, revealing a large abscess of the left breast. The wound was copiously irrigated with antibiotic irrigation and several small areas of oozing were cauterized with Bovie electrocautery. Once the wound was thoroughly cleansed, the wound was reclosed. Hemostasis was meticulously obtained as it was on the day of surgery with Bovie electrocautery. The wound was closed in multiple layers using interrupted inverted Vicryl sutures for the deep dermis and subcutaneous tissues, following which the skin edges were approximated with running subcuticular Monocryl sutures. The nipple–areolar complex was inset in similar fashion. The nipple–areolar complex was viable as it was on the right side. The patient had good shape and symmetry of the breast at the completion of the case.

Identify the physician CPT codes. _____

5. David E.

PREOPERATIVE DIAGNOSIS: Basal cell carcinoma, left nose.
POSTOPERATIVE DIAGNOSIS: 2 × 1 cm basal cell carcinoma, left nose.
PROCEDURE: Excision of basal cell carcinoma.
PREOPERATIVE INDICATIONS: The patient is a 53-year-old man with a history of basal cell cancer of the left scalp. It has now recurred and he is here for excision.
DESCRIPTION OF PROCEDURE: The patient was taken to the operating room and placed in the supine position before induction of anesthesia. The patient was then prepped and draped in the usual sterile fashion. Approximately 7 cc of 1% lidocaine with epinephrine was infiltrated locally. An elliptical incision was made around the 2 cm × 1 cm lesion, affording approximately 2-mm margins. It was carried down full thickness from the skin to the subcutaneous tissue where it was excised with cautery. Tissue was submitted for permanent section.
Bleeding points were cauterized and flaps were raised. Then the 4.5-cm wound was closed with interrupted 4-0 Vicryl in the subcutaneous tissue and 5-0 vertical mattress nylon in the skin.
PATHOLOGY REPORT: Basal cell carcinoma.

Identify the physician CPT codes. _____

6. Charlene M.

PREOPERATIVE DIAGNOSIS: Excess lower abdominal fat and skin with unacceptable cosmetic appearance.
PROCEDURE PERFORMED: Abdominoplasty.
DESCRIPTION OF PROCEDURE: The preoperative markings were made in a semi-upright position in the holding area with a black magic marker, after which photographs were obtained. The patient was then taken to the operating room, where after satisfactory general endotracheal anesthesia was obtained, both arms were well padded and outstretched on arm boards. Bilateral sequential compression stockings were applied and a lower body warming unit was provided. The entire chest and abdomen were then prepped with Betadine solution and draped with sterile drapes, and the lower abdominal incision was then locally anesthetized with an equal volume mixture of 0.5% Marcaine plain diluted with an equal volume of 1% Xylocaine with 1:100,000 epinephrine.

Once adequate local anesthesia and vasoconstriction were obtained, the incision was then carried down through the skin using sharp dissection extending down through the anterior external rectus fascia. The upper abdominal flap was then mobilized. The umbilicus was circumscribed with a #15C blade and the umbilicus was preserved on its normal vascular stalk down to the abdominal wall. The dissection then continued cephalad until the costal margins were visualized. Care was taken to doubly clamp, divide, and ligate the larger musculocutaneous perforators with fine clamps and ligatures of 3-0 Vicryl. Small bleeding points were controlled with electrocautery using a sweetheart retractor. The upper abdominal flap was then elevated and the uppermost portion of the dissection continued with the Bovie electrocautery toward the xiphoid. Once the upper abdominal flap had been mobilized, the rectus abdominis muscles were visualized. There was a slight degree of diastasis rectus, which was then plicated with interrupted figure-of-8 sutures of #0 Ethibond. There was a pleasing improvement in the contour of the musculofascial abdominal wall with no herniation. The wound was then irrigated with copious amounts of bacitracin antibiotic irrigation. The flap was then advanced after gently flexing the operating table. The excess fat–skin apron was then, in a tailor-tacked fashion, sequentially excised, and the upper abdominal flaps were sequentially advanced using a differential suturing technique with interrupted deep fascial and dermal sutures of 2-0 and 3-0 Monocryl, training out the lateral dog ears toward the central portion and minimizing the tension on the skin closure between the medial groin, bilaterally alleviating tension on the mons pubis. Interrupted deep dermal sutures of 4-0 Monocryl were then placed. Sterile extension tubing was placed in the subcutaneous wound toward the xiphoid and brought out through the incision. The new umbilicus was then brought out through a U-shaped skin flap that was created at the same level of the previous umbilicus. A 2-0 PDS suture was placed through the 12 o'clock portion of the new umbilicus through the 6 o'clock portion of the U-shaped flap and through the anterior rectus sheath, creating an inverted umbilicus. Again, there was excellent hemostasis. The PDS layer closure having been effected, the skin edges were then approximated with running 4-0 Monocryl sutures. 30 cc of 0.5% Marcaine plain was then instilled into the operative wound and the catheter was withdrawn.

Identify the physician CPT codes. _____

7. Graciela M.

PREOPERATIVE DIAGNOSIS: Bilateral hypomastia.

PROCEDURE PERFORMED: Bilateral breast augmentation using Mentor style 68 smooth-wall, saline-filled implants: The right breast is filled to 385 cc; the left breast filled to 400 cc.

INDICATIONS FOR PROCEDURE: The patient is a 34-year-old white female who presents with breast hypoplasia. The patient is seeking to increase her breast size to a size and shape that she feels is appropriate for her body habitus.

PROCEDURE: I made an incision on the right breast from 3 o'clock to 9 o'clock along the inferior border of the nipple–areolar complex, dissected through the subcutaneous tissues, and identified the lateral border of the pectoralis major muscle. I elevated the pectoralis major muscle and then proceeded to divide its insertions from the third intercostal space inferiorly and then laterally. I then proceeded to irrigate the pocket copiously with saline and placed a sizer into the pocket. The sizer was inflated to a volume of 375 cc. I then turned her attention to the opposite left breast and performed a mirror image procedure. I removed the sizers and irrigated the pocket with normal saline- and bacitracin-containing solutions. I then proceeded to place the Mentor style 68 implants into position and inflated the left to 400 cc and the right to 385 cc. The patient was brought to the sitting position. I corrected for the patient's breast asymmetries and the higher inframammary crease on the left side, which was lowered. I removed and sealed the fill valves. I used 3-0 Vicryl for deep suture, as well as 4-0 Monocryl and 5-0 Monocryl sutures, and applied one-half-inch Steri-Strips.

Identify the physician CPT codes. _____

8. Steven G.

> **PREOPERATIVE DIAGNOSIS:** Pilonidal cyst with abscess.
>
> **OPERATIVE PROCEDURE:** Excision, curettage, and marsupialization of pilonidal cyst with abscess.
>
> **INDICATIONS:** This 26-year-old man, since autumn, has had at least three flare-ups of an infected pilonidal cyst, which were treated with antibiotics. Typically, the cyst was spontaneously drained once the area was incised. In April, he presented with a painful pilonidal cyst; on examination, he was found to have a 2 cm × 1 cm area of tender erythema with no fluctuance. Distal to that were four pilonidal pits along the intergluteal cleft.
>
> **PATHOLOGICAL FINDINGS:** Examination over the presacral region identified a 2 cm × 1 cm area of erythema and induration with a central punctate opening along the intergluteal cleft, where there were four pilonidal pits. These were approximately 3 cm from the area of erythema. Under the skin was a 6 cm × 1 cm cyst containing granulation tissue and air. There was no evidence of fistula in ano.
>
> **PROCEDURE DESCRIPTION:** A fistula probe was passed into the draining external opening, and the overlying skin was incised along the length of the cyst both in the cephalad and caudal directions. Curettage was performed and all granulation tissue was removed. The cavity was clearly defined, and the overhanging edges of skin and cyst were excised with electrocautery. The fibrous base of the cyst was lightly electrocauterized. The wound was then marsupialized with two continuous 4-0 Vicryl sutures.

Identify the physician CPT codes. _____

9. Stratos P.

> **PREOPERATIVE DIAGNOSIS:** Extensive lipomas of the torso and extremities.
>
> **OPERATIVE PROCEDURE:** Excision of a large lipoma from the left elbow; excision of a lipoma from the left posterior arm.
>
> **INDICATIONS:** This 52-year-old gentleman has perhaps 100 lipomas of his torso and extremities. He presented complaining of pain in some of these lipomas and presents today for excision of the symptomatic lesions.
>
> **PROCEDURE DESCRIPTION:** The patient was taken to the operating room and general anesthesia was administered. The left elbow area was prepped and draped in the usual sterile fashion. A scalpel was used to make an incision overlying the tumor and sharp and blunt dissection was carried through the subcutaneous fat. An 8-cm fatty tumor was removed from the subcutaneous tissue in the elbow area. Skin closure was done with subcuticular Vicryl. The arm was then draped over the chest and the posterior arm was prepped and draped in the usual sterile fashion. Again, a scalpel was used to make a linear incision overlying the tumor. A 10-cm subcutaneous tumor was found, which actually contained multiple lobulated lesions consistent with multiple lipomas. Again, skin closure was done with running subcuticular Vicryl. Sterile dressings were placed over both of these lesions. The arm was placed down at the side. Sterile dressings were applied. The patient was stable and transported to the recovery area.

Identify the physician CPT codes. _____

10. Ralph R.

> **PREOPERATIVE DIAGNOSIS:** Stasis ulcers of the right lower extremity.
> **OPERATION:** Split-thickness skin grafting of a total area of approximately 200 sq. cm on the right leg.
> **INDICATIONS:** This 70-year-old male presented recently with a large ulcer of the lower right leg consistent with a stasis ulcer.
> **PROCEDURE:** Having obtained adequate general endotracheal anesthesia, the patient was prepped from the pubis to the toes. The leg was examined and the wound was Pulsavaced with 2 liters of saline with Bacitracin. The wound was then inspected and there was adequate hemostasis and only minimal fibrinous debris that needed to be removed. Once this was accomplished, the skin graft of 200 sq. cm was harvested from the right thigh and then stapled into position on the wound. The wound was then dressed with a fine mesh gauze that was stapled into position as well as Kerlix soaked in Sulfamylon solution.
> The donor site was dressed with Op-Site. The patient tolerated the procedure well and returned to the recovery room in satisfactory condition.

Identify the physician CPT codes. _____

INTERNET RESEARCH

Search CMS's website www.cms.gov/ for LCDs for benign skin lesion removal. Will the carrier cover removal of a lesion if it shows signs of inflammation?

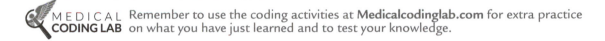 Remember to use the coding activities at **Medicalcodinglab.com** for extra practice on what you have just learned and to test your knowledge.

CPT: Musculoskeletal System

Chapter 18 in *Conquer Medical Coding* focuses on the procedural coding of surgical cases involving problems of the musculoskeletal system. Musculoskeletal codes make up the largest subsection of the CPT Surgery section, because many different procedures can be performed on the bones, tendons, soft tissue, and muscles of the body. These codes are primarily used by emergency department (ED) physicians, urgent care centers, and orthopedic surgeons. Orthopedics (alternate spelling is orthopaedics) deals with prevention and treatment of injuries and diseases of the musculoskeletal system. Correct code assignment in this section is dependent upon the coder being able to determine if the treatment provided is for a traumatic injury (accident) or a medical condition. In addition to explaining the steps for correct coding, the chapter explains the following:

- The organization of the musculoskeletal surgery codes in CPT
- Common musculoskeletal system surgical techniques
- When to use modifiers when coding orthopedic services
- How to determine intraoperative services and imaging guidance work for orthopedic procedures and knowing when they are separately reportable

CODE IT!

Assign all pertinent procedure codes, modifiers, and HCPCS codes.

1. _____ A closed treatment of an ulnar shaft fracture

2. _____ An open treatment of a fractured big toe and application of a short leg cast

3. _____ Arthroscopic chondroplasty of the medial compartment and meniscectomy of the lateral compartment of the right knee

4. _____ I&D of hematoma, right elbow joint

5. _____ Morton's neuroma removal, left foot

6. _____ Left knee arthroscopy with medial and lateral meniscectomy

7. _____ A patient who broke his left arm 4 weeks ago comes in today to have his cast removed and replaced with a short-arm cast

8. _____ Excision of a ganglion cyst of the right foot

9. _____ Closed treatment of ankle dislocation in the ED under conscious sedation

10. _____ Dislocated left patella

MULTIPLE CHOICE

Select the option that best provides the correct code, completes the statement, or answers the question.

1. What is the correct way to code a posterior lumbar arthrodesis, L3–L5?
   A. 22614x3
   B. 22612x2
   C. 22600
   D. 22612, 22614

2. What is the correct way to code for screws placed posteriorly in pedicles of L3 and L5, and attached to a rod that runs from L3 to L5? (All answers are add-on codes.)
   A. 22842, 22841
   B. 22845
   C. 22840
   D. 22840x3

3. Arthrodesis is performed using a metal cage; a hole is drilled in the interspace and a metal cage is placed in the hole. Another metal cage is placed in the same interspace and filled with an autogenous, morselized bone graft from a separate incision. Code for the application of the metal cages and the bone graft.
   A. 22851, 20937–51
   B. 22851x2, 20937–51
   C. 22851
   D. 22851, 20937

4. Standard medial and inferior lateral portals were established. Diagnostic arthroscopy was carried out. The menis was contoured back medially and laterally and chondroplasty performed on the lateral tibial plateau. The patellofemoral joint was inspected and chondroplasty was performed on the under surface of the patella. A lateral retinacular release was performed. What is the correct way to code this situation?
   A. 29870, 29881, 27425–51, 29877–59
   B. 29881, 29873–51, 29877–59
   C. 29870–59, 29880, 29873–51, 29879–59
   D. 29880, 29873–51, 29877–59

5. In the replantation codes (20802–20838), "complete amputation" means that:
   A. The physician will perform a complete amputation before replanting the anatomical area.
   B. The physician will use these codes to indicate replantation after a complete amputation has occurred.
   C. The physician is completely amputating an already partially amputated anatomical area.
   D. The physician has to use the repair of bones, ligaments, tendons, nerves, and so on, in addition to the replantation codes.

6. If an arthroscopic procedure and an open procedure are performed at the same time:
   A. Then only the open procedure can be billed.
   B. Both can be reported if done on different joints.
   C. Both can be reported if one is a diagnostic scope where the decision to proceed to an open procedure is made.
   D. Both a and b are correct.

7. If the code descriptor of a CPT code includes the phrase "separate procedure":
   A. The procedure is subject to NC edits but can be reported separately with a –59 modifier if performed in a separate area.
   B. It is not payable when it is performed at the same patient encounter as another procedure in an anatomically related area through the same skin incision, orifice, or surgical approach.
   C. Both a and b are correct.
   D. It can be coded separately from other procedures performed in the same anatomical area.

8. Select the correct code for an open reduction and internal fixation of a left zygoma fracture in which the patient had a comminuted left lateral rim fracture, including the zygomatic arch, and the orbital floor appeared intact.
   A. 21356
   B. 21366
   C. 21365
   D. 21355

9. A surgeon repairs the flexor tendon on the right foot 15 days after treatment of the patient's left ankle dislocation. Select the correct code for the tendon repair.
   A. 28200–79
   B. 28200–78
   C. 28208–78
   D. 20208–79

10. A patient underwent a talectomy procedure. Where on the body was this procedure performed?
    A. Elbow
    B. Foot
    C. Knee
    D. Ankle

SHORT ANSWER

Answer the following questions.

1. Can external fixation be reported separately from code 23670? Explain your answer. _____

   _____

   _____

2. The patient suffered a penetrating wound to the chest requiring wound exploration. The patient also suffered a fractured shoulder, which required open treatment of the fracture. What modifier will be appended to the wound exploration code and why? _____

   _____

   _____

3. The patient received four trigger point injections into four muscles. The physician reported code 20553x4. The coder wanted the physician to change it to 20553. Who is correct and why? _____

   _____

   _____

4. Two surgeons performed co-surgery for a spinal fusion and a morselized bone graft. Both surgeons wanted to report the spinal fusion code and the bone graft code with a –62 modifier. Is this correct? Explain your answer. _____

_____

_____

5. A physician reported code 20955 with code 69990. The carrier denied 69990. Was the carrier correct? Explain your answer. _____

_____

_____

6. After performing manipulation of the temporomandibular joints under local anesthesia, the physician reported 21073–50. Is this correct? Explain your answer. _____

_____

_____

7. The surgeon performed anterior arthrodesis of T1–T3 and removed some of the disk to accomplish the arthrodesis. The surgeon reported 22556 and 63075. Is the surgeon correct? Explain your answer. _____

_____

_____

8. A surgeon performed a revision of a total hip replacement and reported 27132. Is that correct? Explain your answer. _____

_____

_____

9. A patient had an open repair of a fractured femur and a cast was placed on the leg. Forty-five days later the cast was taken off and a new cast was placed. The office coder instructed the physician that the replacement cast cannot be reported because it is included in the fracture care. Is the coder correct? Explain your answer. _____

_____

_____

10. Code for the application of a multiplane unilateral external fixation system. _____

_____

CASE STUDIES

1. Mathew J.

   Mathew suffers from bursitis and elected to have a steroid injection of the right shoulder. At the physician's office in the minor procedure room, the physician injected Mathew's shoulder with a steroid and anesthetic mixture.

   Assign the code for this procedure. _____

2. Niki D.

Niki is an avid golfer and suffers from medial epicondylitis. Her right elbow is painful and slightly swollen. The pain has worsened despite icing and Advil. A cortisone injection is recommended with use of a sling for 2 weeks. Niki's right elbow was topically anesthetized with ethyl chloride. Under aseptic technique, a 22-G needle was inserted into the soft tissue ending at the tendon origin of the right medial epicondyle. Lidocaine and triamcinolone hexacetonide was injected into the joint without complication.

Assign the code for this procedure. _____

3. Aretha E.

> **FINDINGS AND INDICATIONS:** This 41-year-old white female had a right foot progressively painful over the dorsum at the midfoot area of the joint. She had a progressively enlarging mass. X-rays revealed an osteophyte. We elected to proceed with excision.
> At the time of surgery, there was a fairly large old ganglion cyst underneath hypertrophic bone. The cyst was removed and the hypertrophic bone shaved.
> **PREOPERATIVE and POSTOPERATIVE DIAGNOSIS:** Mass of dorsum of right foot.
> **OPERATION:** Excision of mass right foot (ganglion on top of osteophyte).
> **PROCEDURE:** The patient was taken to the operating room; after satisfactory ankle block anesthesia, the right leg was prepped and draped in a sterile manner. A dorsal incision was made over the mass. The skin and subcutaneous tissue were carefully divided down, looking for the neurovascular bundles. It appeared to be on the lateral side. This was dissected free and retracted lateral.
> A fairly large ganglion cyst was circumferentially resected, then freed. A small stalk went down to an osteophyte. The ganglion was excised and then a rongeur used to remove the stalk. A fairly large osteophyte was also present centrally and then one more on the lateral side. This was removed with a rongeur.
> Final inspection revealed no further prominence. Closure was effected with 4-0 nylon and a pressure dressing was applied.

Code for the procedure. _____

4. Casper G.

> **POSTOPERATIVE DIAGNOSIS:** Two small chondral defects of the medial femoral condyle.
> **OPERATION:** Diagnostic arthroscopy with synovectomy for plica.
> **PROCEDURE:** After satisfactory general endotracheal anesthesia had been obtained, a tourniquet was placed on the left thigh over soft Webril padding.
> The arthroscope was introduced into the knee, which was distended with irrigant. The medial portal was created using a spinal needle for localization. The medial meniscus was examined and found to be intact to visualization and probing. There was a soft strandlike plica from the notch toward the anterolateral portal site, which was resected using a full-radius shaver. The remainder of the knee was then scoped in systematic fashion. The meniscus was found to be stable to visualization and probing. The knee was then irrigated. The arthroscope was withdrawn.

Code for the procedure. _____

5. Oriana L.

> **POSTOPERATIVE DIAGNOSIS:** Discoid lateral meniscus left knee.
>
> **OPERATION:** Arthroscopy left knee with partial lateral meniscectomy left knee.
>
> **PROCEDURE:** The patient's left lower extremity was examined under anesthesia at which time he was found to have no gross ligamentous instability. The left lower extremity was then prepped and draped in normal sterile fashion.
>
> A #11 blade was then used to make an inferolateral arthroscopic portal. The scope was placed in the suprapatellar pouch. The scope was then placed in the intercondylar notch, at which time the anterior and posterior cruciate ligaments were noted to be intact and stable. The scope was then taken into the lateral compartment of the knee, at which time the lateral femoral condyle was noted to be intact. However, the patient did appear to have a discoid lateral meniscus with a small tear at the posterior horn of the lateral meniscus. At that time, a portion of the meniscus was removed, and the knee was then thoroughly irrigated using arthroscopic irrigation. The arthroscopic instruments were removed from the knee. The arthroscopic portals were injected with 0.25% Marcaine with epinephrine, approximately 30 cc into the subcutaneous tissue, followed by 10 cc of Duramorph intra-articularly.

Code for the procedure. _____

6. Jedrek P.

> **PREOPERATIVE DIAGNOSIS:** Left rotator cuff tear.
>
> **POSTOPERATIVE DIAGNOSIS:** Left rotator cuff tear, 6-cm avulsive-type supraspinatus or infraspinatus.
>
> **OPERATION:** Left shoulder arthroscopy, repair rotator cuff.
>
> **PROCEDURE:** The patient was placed in a beach chair with 10 lb. of distraction. Three portals were created anteriorly, laterally, and posteriorly, and the 3M pump was utilized.
>
> The glenohumeral joint revealed that there was at least a tear to the supraspinatus and infraspinatus measuring 6 cm crescent-type supraspinatus or infraspinatus and stellate tear. The articular surfaces were normal. There was a type I labral tear that was debrided; however, there was no biceps tendon tear, and the subscapularis was intact.
>
> The rotator cuff was repaired anatomically after doing an extended portal: first side-to-side with fiberwire #2 back to the tuberosity using three Spiral Locs anchors and #2 Orthocord and Krakow sutures. All knots were very secure and stable with completion while the shoulder was taken through the range of motion.

Code for the procedure. _____

7. Laura V.

> **POSTOPERATIVE DIAGNOSIS:** Left sacroiliitis.
>
> **OPERATIVE PROCEDURE:** Left sacroiliac joint injection under fluoroscopy.
>
> **PROCEDURE DESCRIPTION:** Under fluoroscopy, right oblique view left SI joint was visualized. Corresponding skin entry sites were marked and infiltrated with 0.5 cc of 1% lidocaine. Then, a 3.5-inch-long 25-gauge spinal needle was inserted and advanced under standard fluoroscopy guidance to enter the sacroiliac joint in the lower one-third. After negative aspiration, 1.5-cc solution was injected and made by 40 mg of Depo-Medrol and 0.5 cc of 0.5% Marcaine. The needle was then removed and the skin was cleaned. A Band-Aid was applied.

Code for the procedure. _____

8. Padmaja A.

POSTOPERATIVE DIAGNOSIS: Hallux valgus deformity right foot.
OPERATION: McBride bunionectomy.
PROCEDURE: Pneumatic cuff was placed above the right ankle and after appropriate intravenous sedation had been administered a Mayo-type block was performed using 10 cc of 5% Marcaine solution, plain. The patient was then prepped and draped in the usual aseptic technique. The leg was elevated to allow proper venous drainage. The cuff was inflated to 250 mmHg. The leg was placed back on the operating table and the following procedure was then performed: McBride bunionectomy, right foot. A dorsal linear incision was made medial and parallel to the long extensor tendon centering at the first metatarsal phalangeal joint. The incision was deepened. Superficial vessels were Bovied. Continuous dissection was performed down to the area of the capsule where a linear incision was made and the soft tissue structures were dissected free about the head of the first metatarsal and base of the proximal phalanx. Using a sagittal bone saw, the dorsal and medial redundant bone were removed. The raw bone was rasped smooth; the area was then lavaged with lactated Ringer's and suctioned.

Code for the procedure. _____

9. Delbert F.

PREOPERATIVE DIAGNOSIS: Ruptured right small finger extensor tendon at the DIP joint.
OPERATION: Repair of extensor tendon, right small finger.
PROCEDURE: A dorsal incision was made over the DIP in the right small finger. The extensor tendon was identified and found to be loose medially but especially laterally. Figure-of-eight cinching sutures of 000 Ethibond were placed both medially and laterally along the extensor tendon; this placed the patient in about 10 degrees of hyperextension. The incision was closed with horizontal mattress sutures of 5-0 nylon.

Code for the procedure. _____

10. Shawn G.

POSTOPERATIVE DIAGNOSIS: Delayed union bimalleolar fracture of the right ankle.
OPERATION: Open treatment of bimalleolar fracture of the right ankle.
PROCEDURE: Through a longitudinal incision directed over the lateral aspect of the ankle and distal fibular area, the incision was carried down through skin and subcutaneous tissue. By subperiosteal dissection, the fracture site was identified. The fracture site was reduced by traction and plate and screws were attached to the lateral fibular cortex with an oblique screw across the fracture site from the anterior to posterior plane. Postoperative internal fixation films revealed overall satisfactory fracture and internal fixation appliance positioning. The wound was then packed open with wet Ray-Tec and attention was directed to the medial aspect of the ankle. The incision was carried down through skin and subcutaneous tissue. The fracture site was fibrotic, we elected to reduce the fracture and internally fixate it. The fracture was reduced. A smooth c-wire was inserted across the fracture site. Post pin fixation, x-rays revealed overall satisfactory pin placement, and we proceeded with compression screw fixation. A second drill hole was made through the drill guide anterior to the smooth c-wire and a 50-mm compression screw was inserted across the fracture site. The wound was irrigated and then closed in layers.

Code for the procedure. _____

INTERNET RESEARCH

1. Visit *Coding Coach* at www.karenzupko.com/resources and select the Orthopaedic link. Choose the Coding Coach option and select Orthopaedic. Review the question and answer provided. Do you agree? Is there anything you would change?
2. Visit *OrthoInfo* at http://orthoinfo.aaos.org/main.cfm and search for "Rotator cuff repair." Review the information and answer this question: What are the three most common techniques for rotator cuff repair?

MEDICAL CODING LAB — Remember to use the coding activities at **Medicalcodinglab.com** for extra practice on what you have just learned and to test your knowledge.

CPT: Respiratory System

Chapter 19 in *Conquer Medical Coding* explains the coding and terminology of surgical cases involving procedures within the otorhinolaryngology and pulmonology specialties. Otorhinolaryngology is a surgical subspecialty that concentrates on the diseases and medical and surgical treatments of diseases related to the nose, sinuses, ears, and throat (pharynx and larynx). Pulmonology is a medicine subspecialty that concentrates solely on the medical and minor surgical treatment of the trachea and lungs.

Code assignment requires careful review of the procedural and operative note to determine:
1. The extent of the procedure. To capture all services rendered, the coder must know the anatomical landmarks to recognize when the surgeon has moved to a different structure
2. The technique or approach (open or closed [endoscopic]) the surgeon used
3. The type of procedure—whether it is diagnostic or surgical in nature
4. Whether the procedure was unilateral or bilateral
5. Whether the procedure is considered a component of another major procedure. Surgeries are commonly reported with several CPT codes for each procedure performed

In addition, Chapter 19 explains the following topics:
- The anatomical structures of the nose, sinuses, trachea, larynx, and lungs
- The purpose of the common procedures on the lower respiratory system: laryngoscopy, tracheostomy, bronchoscopy, thoracoscopy, and thoracentesis
- The different codes for nasal and septal fracture repairs, depending on technique, type of fracture, and age of fracture
- The components of a sinus endoscopy
- The differences between various endoscopic sinus procedure codes and how to report multiple surgeries at the same session
- When it is appropriate to separately report image guidance when performed with sinus endoscopies
- The difference between turbinate excision, reduction, and submucous resection and when these are appropriate to report

- When to assign laryngectomy codes when performed with pharyngectomy or radical or modified neck dissection
- The distinction between the various pharyngectomy codes and the correct coding based on the technique applied
- The distinction between lung wedge resection, lobectomy, segmentectomy, and pneumonectomy procedures
- The three components of work for lung transplantation and the appropriate codes to assign for each

CODE IT!

Assign all pertinent procedure codes and modifiers.

1. _____ How would you bill for bilateral sinus endoscopy with removal of tissue from the frontal sinuses and bilateral submucous resection of inferior turbinates?

2. _____ The previous patient needs an endoscopic sinus debridement in the office, 1 week after surgery. How would you bill for this visit?

3. _____ The physician performs a left endoscopic partial ethmoidectomy with left maxillary sinus antrostomy.

4. _____ The patient is scheduled for transbronchial needle aspiration biopsy with fluoroscopic guidance for a lung mass. Following administration of anesthesia, the patient develops atrial fibrillation and the physician elects to terminate the procedure before the biopsy is obtained. How is this coded by the facility?

5. _____ Following general anesthesia, a rigid bronchoscope is inserted and advanced through the larynx to the main bronchus. The area of stenosis is treated with laser therapy.

6. _____ The patient suffers from chronic sinusitis and nasal congestion. The physician performs an endoscopic left anterior and posterior ethmoidectomy with right sphenoidotomy.

7. _____ The patient was involved in a karate match and received a severe kick to the chest. The patient developed breathing problems, and following x-rays the patient was diagnosed with traumatic pneumothorax. A thoracentesis was performed.

8. _____ The patient is diagnosed with a suspicious tumor in the main bronchus. Following general anesthesia, a flexible bronchoscope is inserted and advanced into the main bronchus and the tumor is excised.

9. _____ The patient returns to the doctor's office after having a right side epistaxis packed earlier in the day at his office. The posterior nasal passage is again hemorrhaging and requires packing.

10. _____ The patient is diagnosed with pulmonary alveolar proteinosis and requires total bronchoalveolar lung lavage. A bronchoscope was placed into the left lung and 16 liters of saline was infused.

MULTIPLE CHOICE

Select the option that best provides the correct code, completes the statement, or answers the question.

1. What is the correct way to code for septoplasty for deviated septum?
   A. 30465
   B. 30520
   C. 30465–50
   D. 30620

2. What is the correct way to code for ethmoid sinus resected endoscopically–anterior?
   A. 31254
   B. 31255
   C. 31231
   D. 31255–50

3. What is the correct way to code for endoscopic creation of an opening in the maxillary sinus (antrostomy)?
   A. 31256
   B. 31267
   C. 31233
   D. 31237

4. The patient had a chest x-ray, showing an ill-defined mass. A diagnostic bronchoscopy was performed with a specimen taken of the mass. Pathology finding was positive for cancer and a lobectomy was performed the following week. Disregard the time frame and provide codes for both procedures. Do not code for the x-ray.
   A. 31625, 32480
   B. 31622, 32480
   C. 31625, 32482
   D. 31622, 32482

5. What is the correct code for a sinus endoscopy with anterior and posterior ethmoidectomy?
   A. 31254
   B. 31254–50
   C. 31255
   D. 31255-22

6. What is the correct code for excision of extensive nasal polyps in the hospital setting?
   A. 30115
   B. 30115–22
   C. 30110
   D. 30110–22

7. What is the correct code for bilateral intranasal maxillary sinusotomy (antrostomy)?
   A. 31233–50
   B. 31233
   C. 31256
   D. 31020–50

8. The term *esophagomyotomy* is defined as:
   A. Exploration of the chest muscle
   B. Incision into the muscle of the esophagus
   C. Exploration of the muscle of the esophagus
   D. Incision into the chest muscle

9. A patient with chronic sphenoidal sinusitis has a bilateral sinusotomy. The physician takes a biopsy of the sphenoidal masses and removes the mucosa with several polyps. Transseptal sutures are placed and the intraoral incision is closed in a single layer. The nose is packed and external nasal dressings are placed. What is the correct way to code for this procedure?
   A. 31002
   B. 31002–50
   C. 31051–50
   D. 31051

10. The patient has a large, unresectable right upper lobe mass, suspicious for metastasis. Under fluoroscopic guidance, a percutaneous needle biopsy of the lung lesion is performed for histopathology and tumor markers.
    A. 32405
    B. 32405, 77002
    C. 32098
    D. 32098, 77002

SHORT ANSWER

Answer the following questions.

1. Placement of a scope into the larynx to be viewed via a mirror is defined as: _____

   _____

   _____

2. A surgeon performs an emergency tracheostomy via the cricothyroid membrane for a patient in the ED with crushing injuries suffered in a car accident. What is the correct code for this procedure? _____

   _____

3. Can the codes 31622 and 31629 be reported together? Explain why. _____

   _____

   _____

4. Thoracentesis was performed on the left side of the chest, code 32554. An indwelling tunneled pleural catheter with cuff, code 32550, was placed on the right side. Can both codes be reported together? Explain why. _____

   _____

   _____

5. Why is code 36201 considered bilateral? _____

   _____

   _____

6. A right bilobectomy was performed on a patient 8 months ago. The patient's lung cancer has returned and all of the remaining lung on the right must be removed. What is the correct code for this procedure? _____

   _____

7. What is the code for a total ethmoidectomy performed intranasally? _____

   _____

8. A patient was admitted to the hospital for excision of extensive nasal polyps bilaterally. What is the correct code for this procedure? _____

   _____

9. What anatomical site is defined as the space between the lining of the outside of the lungs and the wall of the chest? _____

   _____

10. The goal of a functional endoscopic sinus surgery is to open which anatomical structure? ___

    _____

CASE STUDIES

1. Aurora M.

   Aurora, a 45-year-old female patient, was brought to the ED by her boyfriend who said she fell in her backyard and was injured in her chest by a sharp object that was sticking up from the ground. The ED physician examined the wound and further dissected it to determine the wound's depth and whether or not there was a foreign object in the wound. He suspected some foreign object remnant and performed an exploratory thoracotomy to determine if anything remained in the chest cavity. Nothing was found and the patient's wound was closed.

   Code for the procedure(s). _____

   _____

2. Charles T.

   > **PREOPERATIVE DIAGNOSIS:** 3-cm carcinoma of the right lower lobe.
   > **PROCEDURE:** Thoracoscopic single lobectomy.
   > Charles, a 70-year-old male smoker, presents with a 3-cm carcinoma in the right lower lobe. Charles is anesthetized, a trocar is inserted, and the thoracoscope is advanced into the pleural cavity. Pleural fluid is sent for cytology and microbiology, and the pulmonary artery is identified and dissected free. The right lower lobe is resected endoscopically and placed in a sterile bag. The specimen is sent to pathology.

   Code for the procedure(s). _____

   _____

3. Tara B.

   Tara, a 68-year-old female patient, has developed worsening dyspnea resulting from pulmonary infiltrates of the right lung. Previous bronchoscopy washings did not produce a diagnosis. She has been admitted for an open lung biopsy via wedge resection of the right lung. An anterolateral thoracotomy incision is made. The chest and lung are explored and abnormalities are noted visually. The area to be biopsied is exposed and a wedge resection is performed, removing the portion of the lung containing both abnormal and normal tissue. A lung specimen is sent to pathology for a frozen section.

   Code for the procedure(s). _____

   _____

4. Collin W.

   Collin is an 18-year-old male who has had a history of cough and recurrent chest infections since early childhood. A clinical diagnosis of generalized bronchiectasis was made last year. Following high resolution CT scanning, the radiologist suggested a diagnosis of diffuse bronchiolitis. There is no history of asthma-like attacks. He was admitted recently for thoracotomy and a wedge resection was performed on the right middle lobe. The right upper and lower lobes (abnormal on CT) were normal on inspection and palpation.

   Code for the procedure(s). _____

   _____

5. Sang-Ook K.

   Sang-Ook, a 79-year-old man with a 50 pack/year smoking history and continued moderate alcohol use, presented to the clinic with a 6-month history of progressive hoarseness, new onset dysphagia, a 20-lb weight loss, chronic cough, and dyspnea. CT scanning from that visit delineated a large right piriform sinus lesion with invasion of the thyroid cartilage. He was staged as a T4 N1 M0 squamous cell carcinoma of the piriform sinus. The patient underwent total laryngectomy and right radical neck dissection.

Code for the procedure(s). _____

_____

6. Fred G.

Fred, a 60-year-old male, was involved in a car accident. An ambulance was called because he developed breathing problems. Upon arrival to the ED, an emergency transtracheal tracheostomy was performed through a horizontal neck incision, dissecting the muscles to expose the trachea. The trachea was incised and an airway was inserted.

Code for the procedure(s). _____

_____

7. Sam S.

PREOPERATIVE DIAGNOSIS: Dysphagia and upper airway obstruction.
OPERATION: Nasal septoplasty.
PROCEDURE: There was marked septal deformity noted, predominantly to the patient's right side, and lower turbinate engorgement was identified bilaterally. A left incision was then utilized to gain access to the submucoperichondrial and mucoperiosteal layers of the nasal septum. The inferior aspect of the anterior cartilaginous septum was then trimmed so as to relocate this to the midline. The posterior deflected portions of the quadrangular cartilage were removed and scored so as to straighten it.

Code for the procedure(s). _____

_____

8. Katie N.

PREOPERATIVE DIAGNOSIS: Persistent epistaxis.
OPERATION: Nasal endoscopy with cauterization.
PROCEDURE: The nose was examined, the endoscope was inserted, and the nasal passages were suctioned of blood clots. With very minimal suction trauma, very brisk bleeding occurred from an arteriole on the left floor of the nose. The arteriole was cauterized. A similar arteriole on the right side also bled with a pumping type of bleeding; again, the arteriole was cauterized on the right. The nose was carefully examined again and no additional bleeding sites were identified.

Code for the procedure(s). _____

_____

9. Constance V.

After discovery of a pleural lesion, the physician performs a percutaneous needle biopsy of the pleura with fluoroscopic guidance. The physician punctures through the chest tissues between two ribs. The needle enters the pleural cavity and slightly punctures the surface of the lung and withdraws a piece of tissue. The puncture site is covered with a bandage.

Code for the needle biopsy. _____

_____

10. Evan A.

Evan, a 2-year-old child, presents to his pediatrician's office after his mother notices a foul odor coming from the child's nose and suspects that Evan has put one of the buttons from her sewing kit into his nose. Topical and local anesthesia is applied to the nasal mucosa. The button is retrieved with forceps.

Code for the procedure(s). _____

_____

INTERNET RESEARCH

1. Visit the American Academy of Otolaryngology—Head and Neck Surgery's Coding Corner at http://www.entnet.org/content/coding-cornerClick on Practice Management. Under Resources select either Coding Corner and pick a topic under Coding Guidance: CPT for ENT Articles and Code Changes/Edits, or Clinical Practice Guidelines, or Reimbursement and present this to your class.
2. Visit the American Thoracic Society's Clinical Resources web page at www.thoracic.org/professionals/clinical-resources/. On the left is a link for ATS clinical cases, select that link and scroll down the list to "Incidental pulmonary nodule in a 75 year old man" and code for the surgery.

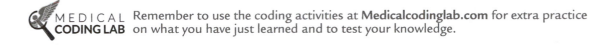 Remember to use the coding activities at **Medicalcodinglab.com** for extra practice on what you have just learned and to test your knowledge.

CPT: Cardiovascular, Hemic, and Lymphatic Systems

Chapter 20 in *Conquer Medical Coding* explains the steps in selecting codes for the most common arterial, venous, and lymphatic procedures, as well as the major heart procedures, such as coronary artery bypass grafts and the interventional cardiovascular procedures. For cardiovascular procedures especially, a coder must be sure to understand the terminology and where in the cardiovascular system the procedure is being performed, as well as how many codes are needed. Potentially, a coder could be assigning codes from three different sections of the CPT book. The chapter also explains the following:

- The anatomical structures of the cardiovascular, hemic, and lymphatic systems and their purpose
- The concept of component coding
- The most common abbreviations and acronyms used in cardiovascular coding
- The three methods of coronary artery bypass procedures
- The five vascular systems and the concept of vascular families
- The difference between endovascular versus open cardiovascular procedures
- The difference between a pacemaker and cardioverter defibrillator
- The three types of services in heart transplants

CODE IT!

Assign all pertinent procedure codes, modifiers, and HCPCS codes.

1. _____ There is wound dehiscence at the patient's pacemaker site; it requires revision of the site with reinsertion of the single-chamber pulse generator.

2. _____ The cardiologist removes the old pulse generator and inserts a new generator and a new left ventricular electrode.

3. _____ The patient with a history of heart block now requires a dual-chamber pacemaker system. The previous system was single chamber. The pulse generator is removed, the atrial electrode remains in place, and a new ventricular electrode is added.

4. _____ A patient with breast cancer is now undergoing complete axillary lymphadenectomy.

5. _____ An 11-month-old child undergoes a cutdown venipuncture.

6. _____ Subsequent pericardiocentesis is performed with radiological supervision and interpretation.

7. _____ Re-operation is performed for carotid thromboendarterectomy 6 months after the original surgery.

8. _____ The patient is examined because of shortness of breath, and angiography reveals a pulmonary embolus. A surgeon performs an embolectomy of the pulmonary artery. Code for the surgery.

9. _____ After involvement in a motor vehicle accident, the patient suffered blunt trauma rupturing her spleen. The surgeon performed a partial splenectomy.

10. _____ A patient has an infrarenal abdominal aortic and iliac aneurysm that is repaired with an aortic-uni-iliac endograft. Code for the endograft and the RSI.

MULTIPLE CHOICE

Select the option that best provides the correct code, completes the statement, or answers the question.

1. A femoral to popliteal artery in-situ bypass graft is performed with intraoperative angiography. What is the correct way to code this procedure?
   A. 35583, 75820
   B. 35556, 75820
   C. 35556
   D. 35583

2. Because of re-occlusion of a femoral to popliteal bypass graft performed 2 years ago, the surgeon performs a re-operation on the bypass graft with vein. What is the correct way to code this procedure?
   A. 35556, 35700–51
   B. 35556, 35700
   C. 35583, 35700–51
   D. 35583, 35700

3. The cardiologist creates a subclavicular pocket for the pulse generator and inserts a permanent pacemaker with transvenous atrial and ventricular electrodes. What is the correct way to code this procedure?
   A. 33208
   B. 33211
   C. 33202
   D. 33208–62

4. A patient is complaining of sharp, intermittent retrosternal pain that is reduced by sitting up or leaning forward. He is evaluated by his cardiologist who orders a chest x-ray revealing a pericardial effusion. A pericardiocentesis is performed. What is the correct way to code this procedure?
   A. 33010
   B. 33011
   C. 99201, 33010
   D. 99201–25, 33010

5. The patient underwent resection of an intracardiac tumor with cardiopulmonary bypass. What is the correct way to code this procedure?
   A. 33130
   B. 33130, 33141
   C. 33120
   D. 33120, 33141

6. With the heart exposed through the sternum and the patient's functions supported by cardiopulmonary bypass, the right atrium is opened and the supraventricular arrhythmias are ablated by using electrical current. What is the correct way to code this procedure?
   A. 33251
   B. 33249
   C. 33250
   D. 33254

7. A patient has developed occlusive artery disease of the common femoral artery and requires a repair of a pseudoaneurysm with graft insertion. What is the correct way to code this procedure?
   A. 35371
   B. 35141
   C. 35142
   D. 35141, 35142–51

8. After years of heartburn and gastric reflux, a patient undergoes repair of diaphragmatic hernia. What is the correct way to code this procedure?
   A. 39540
   B. 39560
   C. 39541
   D. 39503

9. Code for the bilateral open surgical exposure of the femoral artery for passage of an endovascular sheath to repair an abdominal aortic aneurysm.
   A. 34812
   B. 34812–50
   C. 34800
   D. 34800–22

10. A patient's echocardiogram and cardiac catheterization show severe mitral stenosis with regurgitation. The surgeon performs a mitral valve replacement including cardiopulmonary bypass. What is the correct way to code this procedure?
    A. 33405
    B. 33420
    C. 33425
    D. 33430

SHORT ANSWER

Answer the following questions.

1. A patient with a single-chamber pacemaker now needs a dual-chamber pacemaker. Would the old pulse generator be removed? If so, why? _____

   _____

2. What code would be reported for the insertion of a pacing cardioverter defibrillator? _____

   _____

3. Code for the coronary artery bypass graft of three coronary arteries using the saphenous vein as the graft material. _____

   _____

4. Which, if any, additional code would be needed if the femoropopliteal vein was also used for the bypass graft in question 3? _____

   _____

5. Noncoronary artery bypass grafts are reported three different ways. One is with vein, the second is with other than vein. What is the third? _____

_____

6. Name one of the five vascular systems. _____

7. How many codes are required to report a coronary artery bypass graft using one vein and one artery? _____

8. Name one of the great vessels of the heart. _____

9. The surgeon performed selective catheter placement into the common carotid artery, with radiological supervision and interpretation (RSI). She wants to report 36222, 36221, and the RSI code. The coder explains that the nonselective code 36221 and the RSI code are included in 36222. Is the coder correct? Explain your answer. _____

_____

_____

10. Can CPT code 33210 be reported with code 33256? Explain your answer. _____

_____

_____

CASE STUDIES

1. John P.

> **PREOPERATIVE DIAGNOSIS:** Carotid artery embolus.
> **PROCEDURE:** Embolectomy of the carotid artery.
> **INDICATIONS:** The patient has worked for over 30 years in his restaurant. He recently began fainting during the day but didn't tell anyone until one afternoon when his wife found him passed out on the kitchen floor and called an ambulance. In the ED, a vascular surgeon was called in to evaluate the patient; after testing, it was determined that the patient had an embolus in his carotid artery. An embolectomy of the carotid artery was performed.

Code for the procedure. _____

2. Barbara A.

> **PREOPERATIVE DIAGNOSIS:** Left carotid stenosis.
> **OPERATION:** Left carotid endarterectomy with patch angioplasty.
> After general anesthesia was administered, a left neck incision was made just anterior to the left sternocleidomastoid, which was dissected down to the platysma. High grade stenosis within the internal carotid was noted, which was an acute thrombus; it was removed. The Sachs dissector was then used to perform an endarterectomy. An 8-mm woven Dacron graft was then used to provide a patch to that area.

Code for the procedure. _____

3. Harold W.

PREOPERATIVE DIAGNOSIS: Aortic valve stenosis.
OPERATION: Aortic valve replacement.
The aorta was opened and examined. There were heavy calcifications at the right coronary annulus, and the valve was thickened with some calcific changes, which were worse on the anterior part of the aortic valve. The valve was excised and calcium was debrided carefully. Sutures were placed from the aorta to the ventricular side and a 21-mm AHP aortic valve was inserted in place. Plegia was administered. The incision was closed.

Code for the procedure. _____

4. Vera A.

PREOPERATIVE DIAGNOSIS: Right leg ischemia.
PROCEDURES: Revascularization of right common iliac artery with stent.
INDICATIONS FOR PROCEDURE: This 65-year-old woman presented with right leg ischemia yesterday and underwent right iliac angioplasty and stent. At the time of this procedure, her right common iliac artery was noted to have some stenosis present, about 70% to 80%. She comes to the operating room for revascularization.
DESCRIPTION OF PROCEDURE: The patient was brought into the operating room. General anesthesia was established, and she was prepped and draped in the usual sterile fashion. A right groin longitudinal incision was made, and right common femoral artery and superficial femoral artery were dissected out. A guidewire was advanced into the abdominal aorta and a catheter was advanced proximally into the distal abdominal aorta.
Next, an 18-mm balloon was selected and advanced through the left groin into the aortic bifurcation. The stent was selected and placed at the right common iliac artery and deployed.

Code for the procedure. _____

5. Phyllis J.

PREOPERATIVE DIAGNOSIS: Thrombosis of left above-the-knee femoral-popliteal polytetrafluoroethylene graft.
PROCEDURES: Left femoral-popliteal graft thrombectomy; intraoperative angiography.
DESCRIPTION OF PROCEDURE: The patient's left leg was prepped and draped in the usual sterile fashion. The femoral artery was identified; control of the common femoral, superficial femoral, and deep femoral, as well as the graft, was gained. There was no pulse in the graft.
A graftotomy was performed with an 11-blade scalpel, which was extended with Potts scissors. There appeared to be a clot within the lumen. A #4 Fogarty catheter was passed to this, and there was a good common femoral pulse. The Fogarty catheter was then passed down distally, and a significant amount of clot was brought out from the graft. The graft was then injected with heparinized saline multiple times. There was only a mild amount of back-bleeding. There was excellent bleeding through the graft.
An 8-French introducer catheter was then placed into the graft, and an arteriogram was then performed. It showed that the graft was completely patent, and that the distal anastomosis was patent. The graftotomy was then closed with 5-0 Gortex suture.

Code for the procedure. _____

6. Anil S.

PREOPERATIVE DIAGNOSIS: Severe coronary artery disease with unstable angina.
OPERATION: Coronary artery bypass graft.
INDICATIONS: This 57-year-old patient underwent evaluation for severe coronary disease. Catheterization demonstrates severe coronary disease with a subtotal right coronary artery. Ventricular function was preserved.
DESCRIPTION OF PROCEDURE: While in the supine position under general anesthesia, the patient was prepped and draped in standard fashion. Saphenous vein was taken from the right leg, and this wound was closed in routine fashion. Simultaneously, the chest was opened through a median sternotomy.
We then opened the pericardium and heparinized and cannulated the aorta and right atrium. We went on bypass and cooled down. The aorta was cross-clamped and cardioplegia was infused in the root. We then bypassed the right coronary artery just beyond the acute angle of the heart. It was about 2.0 mm. The aortic cross-clamp was removed and the vein anastomosis was made to the ascending aorta. We weaned from bypass with good hemodynamics. The heart was decannulated, protamine was administered, and hemostasis was obtained. Atrial and ventricular pacing wires were attached and chest tubes were inserted. The mediastinum was copiously irrigated out and it was closed in layers.

Code for the procedure. _____

7. Paige J.

PREOPERATIVE DIAGNOSIS: Laceration of the inferior vena cava.
PROCEDURE: Ligation of the inferior vena cava.
This patient suffered a stab wound to the abdomen, causing injury to the vena cava. The abdomen was explored. Ring forceps and sponges were utilized to occlude blood flow, manually compressing the vena cava. The vena cava was exposed and soft tissue dissected from the surface of the vena cava. The determination was made that the vena cava could not be repaired and ligation was required. The suture ligation was applied to the superior and inferior ends of the inferior vena cava controlling the hemorrhage. The abdomen was re-explored to ensure there was no additional injury. The laparotomy site was closed.

Code for the procedure. _____

8. Lee A.

PREOPERATIVE DIAGNOSIS: Occlusion left common femoral artery.
OPERATION: Left common femoral thromboendarterectomy.
PROCEDURE: The patient was taken to the operating room where he was placed supine on the operating room table. General endotracheal anesthesia was established. Next, a vertical incision was made in the patient's left groin approximately 8 cm in length using a #10 blade. Dissection went through the subcutaneous tissues down through the fascia. The left common femoral artery was exposed and dissected free from surrounding tissue. An arteriotomy was made and a 6-French femoral sheath was placed within the lumen of the common femoral artery extending proximally.
At this point in the procedure, an angiogram was performed that showed there was extensive plaque within the common femoral artery in this location. The left common femoral thromboendarterectomy was performed. The arteriotomy was closed using a running 5-0 Prolene suture. The distal clamp was released first followed subsequently by the proximal clamp. The anastomosis appeared to be intact. There was a palpable pulse proximally and distally. The wound was copiously irrigated and closed in two layers using a running 2-0 Vicryl suture and the skin was closed using skin staples. A sterile dressing was applied over the left groin.

Code for the procedure. _____

9. Chau L.

> **PREOPERATIVE DIAGNOSIS:** Descending thoracic aneurysm.
>
> **PROCEDURE:** Repair of descending thoracic aneurysm with 26-mm tube Dacron woven graft.
>
> **INDICATIONS FOR PROCEDURE:** A 64-year-old male with a history of thoracic aneurysm that has grown over the last 6 months.
>
> **PROCEDURE:** The patient was brought to the operating room and placed in a supine position. General anesthesia was administered. The posterolateral thoracotomy incision was made at the level of the fifth intercostal space. The aneurysm was identified. Proximal and distal clamps were placed and the aneurysm was opened longitudinally. The 26-mm Dacron woven graft was brought into the field and proximal and distal anastomoses were performed end-to-end.

Code for the procedure. _____

10. Nathaniel D.

> **PREOPERATIVE DIAGNOSIS:** A 5.5-cm infrarenal abdominal aortic aneurysm.
>
> **PROCEDURES:** Endovascular aneurysm repair with aorto-aortic endograft.
>
> **DESCRIPTION OF PROCEDURE:** After adequate regional anesthesia had been obtained, the patient's abdomen and groin were sterily prepped and draped and a vertical incision was made for about 6 cm overlying the right common femoral artery. This was carried down to the femoral vessels, which were then controlled circumferentially at the common femoral, profunda femoris, and superficial femoral arteries. At that point, a needle and wire were introduced with introducers, then following subsequently a dilator. A pigtail catheter was placed for angiography. Then the graft was introduced into the main body through the open right femoral cutdown and positioned at the level of the left renal artery, which was the inferior of the two. The graft was then deployed and secured in place by several balloon dilations and a completion angiography was done to ensure that there were no endograft leaks. The patient's pulse was ensured. The groin was then closed in three layers of running Vicryl with a Monocryl subcutaneous suture. The patient was taken from the operating room to the recovery room in stable condition without complications.

Code for the procedure. _____

INTERNET RESEARCH

1. Go to http://www.mayoclinic.org and enter "coronary bypass surgery" into the search box. Use the information you find to define coronary bypass surgery and describe the procedure.
2. At the same website, now search for "atrial fibrillation" in the search box. Find the four most common methods to correct atrial fibrillation.

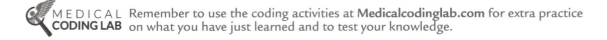 MEDICAL CODING LAB Remember to use the coding activities at **Medicalcodinglab.com** for extra practice on what you have just learned and to test your knowledge.

CPT: Digestive System

Chapter 21 in *Conquer Medical Coding* explains the steps in selecting codes for the most common diseases and disorders of the digestive system and the surgical techniques to treat them. Much of the work done in the digestive system involves endoscopy. The chapter also covers the following:

- The anatomical structures of the lips, mouth, esophagus, stomach, intestines, and anus
- When multiple endoscopy codes can be assigned
- The difference between esophagoscopy and esophagogastroduodenoscopy (EGD)
- The difference between a screening and diagnostic colonoscopy
- The different types of hernias and how they are repaired
- The various bariatric procedures available for weight reduction

CODE IT!

Supply the correct CPT, and HCPCS codes if required, for the following.

1. _____ Proctosigmoidoscopy with laser destruction of polyps

2. _____ Hemorrhoidectomy, internal and external, single column with removal of anal fissures

3. _____ Rigid esophagoscopy with foreign body removal

4. _____ ERCP with removal of pancreatic stones

5. _____ I&D peritonsillar abscess

6. _____ Repair of epigastric strangulated hernia

7. _____ Rectal stricture dilation under general anesthesia

8. _____ Excision of lesion of palate with local flap closure

9. _____ Abdominal and transanal hemicolectomy

10. _____ Salivary gland biopsy by incision

MULTIPLE CHOICE

Select the option that best provides the correct code, completes the statement, or answers the question.

1. A 41-year-old female patient has been experiencing right flank pain radiating to the shoulder and irregular bowel movements. Ultrasound showed a 4+ gallbladder with two large stones. The patient undergoes a laparoscopic cholecystectomy with common bile duct exploration. What code should be reported?
   A. 47562
   B. 47563
   C. 47564
   D. 47579

2. The patient presents with a longstanding history of abdominal pain and now presents with acute rebound tenderness of the right lower quadrant. Exploratory laparotomy with appendectomy is performed. What code(s) should be reported?
   A. 49000, 44955
   B. 49010, 44950
   C. 44970
   D. 44950

3. A 4-year-old boy presents with a bulge in the left inguinal area and an associated hydrocele on examination. The surgeon performs an open inguinal hernia repair with hydrocelectomy. What code(s) should be reported?
   A. 49505, 55500
   B. 49520, 55000
   C. 49495
   D. 49500

4. A 4-year-old swallowed a small toy that got stuck in her throat. A flexible esophagoscopy was performed to remove the toy. What code should be reported?
   A. 43200
   B. 43235
   C. 43247
   D. 43215

5. Assign the appropriate code(s) for EGD with biopsies of the stomach and duodenum and injection of implant material into the muscle of the lower esophageal sphincter.
   A. 43235, 43239
   B. 43239, 43236
   C. 43239, 11900
   D. 43239

6. A 40-year-old male has had severe gastroesophageal reflux disease (GERD) for almost a year. After a previous endoscopy of the esophagus and a barium swallow, the physician determines that he will perform a laparoscopic Nissen procedure. Code for the Nissen procedure.
   A. 3280
   B. 43328
   C. 43327
   D. 43279, 43280–51

7. A 48-year-old man went to the emergency department (ED) complaining of vomiting coffee ground material several times within the past hour. He had abdominal pain and had been unable to eat for the past 24 hours. He was dizzy and lightheaded. His stools today have been black and tarry. While in the ED, he vomited bright red blood and some coffee ground material. After evaluating the patient, a gastrointestinal (GI) consult was requested. The GI physician took the patient to the endoscopy suite and performed an upper GI endoscopy for diagnostic purposes. What code(s) should the GI physician report?
   A. 99245–57, 43235
   B. 43235
   C. 43200, 43235
   D. 43243

8. An endoscope was inserted into the esophagus, and the stomach was entered. The pyloric channel was traversed, showing a pyloric stenosis. The endoscopy was then introduced into the second portion of the duodenum, which showed normal mucosa. A 15-mm balloon was placed across the stenosis and dilated and then withdrawn. What code should be reported?
   A. 43205
   B. 43249
   C. 43204
   D. 43245

9. A diagnostic colonoscopy and a diagnostic EGD are performed on the same patient by the same physician on the same day but not during the same session. Code for both procedures.
   A. 45378, 43235–59
   B. 45378, 43235–51
   C. 45330, 43200–51
   D. 45330, 43200–59

10. The child's gestational age at birth was 34 weeks. Fourteen weeks later, she had an initial inguinal hernia repair done. What code should be reported?
   A. 49491
   B. 49491–63
   C. 49495
   D. 49495–63

SHORT ANSWER

Answer the following questions.

1. A 68-year-old patient is seen for a screening colonoscopy. The patient has been experiencing abdominal pain and diarrhea for the past 6 weeks. He states he has a family history of colon cancer. The colonoscopy was normal and the patient is scheduled for an EGD next week. What code should be reported? _____

_____

2. The patient's esophageal cancer has made it almost impossible for him to eat normally, and he is becoming malnourished. His physician recommends laparoscopically creating an opening into the jejunum (second portion of the small intestine) to allow for placement of a feeding tube. A laparoscopic jejunostomy is performed. What code(s) should be reported? _____

_____

3. As a result of spasms in the esophagus, the patient is unable to swallow food and frequently chokes and needs to regurgitate. At the hospital's GI endoscopy suite, the physician uses a 38-mm balloon dilator to alleviate this patient's difficulty. He uses fluoroscopy to guide placement of the balloon. What code(s) should be reported? _____

_____

4. A patient undergoes a cholecystectomy. During the procedure, an incidental appendectomy is performed. If both procedures are to be reported, what codes should be used?_____

_____

5. The patient has a mass of the soft palate at the left retromolar trigone. The patient is admitted to the ASC to have this mass excised. An incision was made overlying the 1.0-cm cystic mass of the soft palate at the retromolar trigone. By sharp and blunt dissection with the Metzenbaum scissors, the mass was circumferentially dissected from the surrounding tissue and excised en bloc and intact. It was then sent to the pathology department. Bovie was used to cauterize the site and control bleeding, and the site was closed with suture. What code(s) should be reported?_____

_____

6. A toddler is seen in the ED after suspecting he may have ingested an unknown number of Tylenol obtained from a bottle on the counter that was not sealed. To determine if any medicine was in his stomach, the ED physician inserted a nasogastric tube to aspirate contents for specimen testing. No lavage was done yet. What code(s) should be reported?_____

_____

7. The patient was a smoker and smokeless tobacco user. The physician performed resection of a squamous cell carcinoma of the lower lip. A complex, full-thickness repair of the vermilion was also performed. What code(s) should be reported? _____

_____

8. The first steps to choosing the correct endoscopy code are to determine _____ the scope was inserted, whether it is a diagnostic or _____, and the _____ to which the scope was passed.

9. A patient is admitted with hematemesis for suspected bleeding stomach ulcer. EGD is performed to diagnose the cause of the bleeding. An active ulcer was identified and cautery was performed. What code(s) should be reported?_____

_____

10. The patient is morbidly obese with a BMI of 60. He elected to proceed with a laparoscopic gastric bypass to the ileum. What code(s) should be reported?_____

_____

CASE STUDIES

1. Shawn C.

> **PROCEDURE:** Screening colonoscopy with hot biopsy polypectomy.
> **DESCRIPTION OF PROCEDURE:** The patient was placed in the left lateral decubitus position and sedated with a normal amount of monitored anesthesia care (MAC) sedation. The scope was passed easily into the rectum. The scope was passed up to the level of the cecum. In the sigmoid colon at 15 cm, a 2-mm polyp was seen and removed by hot biopsy polypectomy. The scope was withdrawn from the patient.

Assign the CPT procedure code(s) for the physician. _____

2. Fana K.

> **PROCEDURE:** Esophagogastroduodenoscopy with biliary secretion sampling and gastric biopsies.
> **ANESTHESIA:** Fentanyl 50 mg, Versed 3.5 mg administered by nurse anesthetist.
> The patient was taken to the endoscopy suite and placed on the left lateral decubitus position. Her oropharynx was anesthetized with a topical anesthetic, and she was given intravenous sedation. The Olympus flexible video endoscope was introduced under direct visualization into the esophagus without complications. The scope was then advanced through the esophagus and stomach and into the first and second portions of the duodenum. The patient was then given a dose of 1.6 cc of Kinevac. Minimal bile was produced with this. The patient was then given a second dose of 3.2 cc of Kinevac. There was good flow of bile into the duodenum, and approximately 7 to 10 cc were removed for sampling. The scope was then withdrawn. The duodenal bulb was without abnormality. The pylorus was visualized and showed no evidence of ulcer formation. Three biopsies were taken of the antrum to rule out *H pylori*, but there was no evidence of antritis. The GE junction was examined and was normal. The scope was withdrawn to the GE junction. This was at 40 cm. Again, there were no abnormalities at or above the GE junction. The remainder of the esophagus was normal.
> **PATHOLOGY SPECIMEN:** Antral biopsy, r/o *H pylori*.
> **POSTOPERATIVE DIAGNOSIS:** Chronic active gastritis with organisms showing features of *H pylori* identified.

a. *Assign the CPT procedure codes for the physician.* _____

b. *Can the IV conscious sedation be reported separately? If yes, what code is assigned?* _____

_____

3. Hikaru S.

> **AGE:** 67, Medicare patient with no prior colon evaluation.
> **OPERATION:** Screening complete colonoscopy.
> **PROCEDURE:** The patient was taken to the endoscopy suite after administration of IV sedation by the anesthesia department. The patient was positioned in the left lateral decubitus position. The flexible colonoscope was navigated through the anus to 155 cm, at which time the ileocecal valve was identified and verified by light verification and palpation of the right lower quadrant. No tumors, masses, or polyps were seen. Sigmoid diverticulosis was seen. The patient tolerated the procedure well. The scope was withdrawn and no evidence of any tumors or masses was seen in the rectum or perianal area. The patient tolerated the procedure and was sent to the post-procedure area for further monitoring.

Assign the CPT procedure codes for the physician. _____

4. Stannard N.

> **INDICATIONS:** Dysphagia. Intermittent solid food obstruction in his esophagus.
> **PROCEDURE:** The fiber-optic video endoscope was advanced through the patient's mouth and into the esophagus. The esophagus appeared to be within normal limits in the upper two-thirds portion. The distal one-third of the esophagus showed severe mucosal erythema, friability, and erosion. There was early esophageal stricturing present. The stomach showed a moderate-sized sliding hiatal hernia. The gastric mucosa was erythematous and friable throughout. Biopsy was obtained of the antrum and submitted for *Campylobacter*-like organism (CLO) testing. The pylorus and duodenum appeared within normal limits. A spring-tipped guide wire was advanced through the biopsy channel of the endoscope and delivered into the stomach. The endoscope was then withdrawn and the guide wire left in place. Dilators were then passed over the guide wire through the mouth, through the esophagus, and into the stomach. Dilators size 14 mm and then 16 mm were used without difficulty.

a. *What procedure was performed for the esophageal stricture?* _____

_____

b. *Where was the erosion located?* _____

_____

c. *How far was the endoscope advanced?* _____

_____

d. *Assign the CPT procedure codes for the physician.* _____

5. Ray V.

> **OPERATION:**
> 1. Esophagogastroduodenoscopy with biopsy at 40 cm at the EG junction
> 2. Complete colonoscopy
>
> **PROCEDURE:** The patient was taken to the endoscopy suite. After administration of IV sedation by the anesthesia department, the patient was positioned in the left lateral decubitus position. The posterior pharynx was previously anesthetized with Cetacaine spray, and the scope was navigated through a bite block into the posterior pharynx, through to the posterior pharynx into the esophagus, from the esophagus into the stomach, through a patent pylorus, through the first portion into the second portion of the duodenum. No tumors, masses, or outlet obstructions were seen, nor any ulcerations. The scope was withdrawn. There was a small hiatal hernia without any associated complications noted. No strictures, erosions, or varix were identified. A representative area of the EG junction was biopsied at 40 cm. The scope was withdrawn after desufflating the upper GI tract. The proximal esophageal mucosa appeared normal. The scope was removed, and the patient was repositioned on the stretcher.
>
> The flexible colonoscope was navigated through the anus, to 145 cm, at which time the ileocecal valve was identified and verified by light verification and palpation of the right lower quadrant. No tumors, masses, or polyps were seen. No diverticuli or bleeding sites were seen. As the scope was withdrawn, small internal hemorrhoids were identified at the outlet. The patient tolerated the procedure well and was sent to the post-procedure area for further monitoring.

a. *Was a complete colonoscopy performed? How do you know?* _____

_____

_____

b. *Assign the CPT procedure codes for the physician.* _____

6. Auburn G.

> **PREOPERATIVE DIAGNOSIS:** Blood in stool and positive family history of colon cancer.
> **OPERATION:** Complete colonoscopy.
> **PROCEDURE:** The patient was taken to the endoscopy suite after administration of IV sedation by the anesthesia department. The patient was positioned in the left lateral decubitus position. The flexible colonoscope was navigated through the anus to 150 cm, at which time the ileocecal valve was identified and verified by light verification and palpation of the right lower quadrant. No tumors, masses, or polyps were seen. No diverticuli were seen. There were large internal and external hemorrhoids noted at the outlet. The patient tolerated the procedure well. The colon was desufflated. The scope was removed.

a. *Is this a screening colonoscopy?* _____

b. *Assign the CPT procedure codes for the physician.* _____

7. Olaf S.

PROCEDURE PERFORMED: PPH (procedure for prolapse and hemorrhoids—stapled hemorrhoidopexy).

INDICATIONS: On examination, the patient was found to have a moderate-sized edematous left lateral external hemorrhoid with a large prolapse, left lateral internal hemorrhoidal column, containing several small thromboses. The right-sided external hemorrhoids were small. Anoscopy identified multiple groups of large, inflamed internal hemorrhoids.

PROCEDURE DESCRIPTION: The buttocks were taped apart, and the perianal area was prepped and painted with Betadine and sterilely draped. Local anesthesia was infiltrated circumanally and deeper for a bilateral rectal block. The anus was gently and digitally dilated to a finger-breadth. Examination under anesthesia was performed with the previous findings.

A Fansler retractor was placed to expose the field of operation. Beginning posteriorly, a #2-0 Prolene suture was placed in a purse-string fashion along the submucosal plane approximately 4 to 5 cm above the dentate line. Care was taken not to incorporate the underlying rectal vault. When this was completed, the Fansler retractor was removed and the PPH anal canal dilator and obturator were then placed over the purse-string suture and carefully positioned to protect the anal sphincter complex and keep the anoderm out of the field of operation. The PPHO3 stapler was then fully opened and the anvil was placed proximal to the purse-string suture. The purse-string suture was secured around the shaft of the anvil, then retrieved through the barrel of the stapler with a suture threader. The suture was secured upon itself and retracted as the stapler was then fully closed. The 4-cm mark on the barrel of the stapler was just up within the anal wedge, indicating proper positioning. The stapler was kept closed for 30 seconds, fired, released, removed, opened, and inspected. It contained circumferentially complete donor tissue composed of only mucosa and submucosa with no evidence of muscular fat. This was sent to the pathology department.

a. *Is the examination under anesthesia separately reportable?* _____

b. *Can the bilateral rectal block be reported separately?* _____

c. *Assign the CPT procedure codes for the physician.* _____

8. Ellen A.

PROCEDURE PERFORMED: Colonoscopy via the anus and via colostomy.

CLINICAL NOTE: The patient is status post-sigmoid colectomy for perforated sigmoid diverticulitis. She is scheduled for take down of the colostomy tomorrow and presents today for preoperative evaluation with colonoscopy to be certain that the anatomy is acceptable for laparoscopic take down of the colostomy and to rule out stricture, tumor, and so on.

DESCRIPTION OF PROCEDURE: The colonoscope was advanced to the end of the Hartmann pouch and was withdrawn. The Hartmann pouch appears to be fairly straight. The colonoscope was then introduced into the colostomy and advanced all the way to the cecum. The scope was gradually withdrawn through the cecum. The prep was excellent. There was no pathology noted except for the diverticulosis in the left colon.

Assign the CPT procedure codes for the physician. _____

9. Hulda G.

PROCEDURE: Submuscular anal fistulotomy.

OPERATION: A fistula probe was gently used to examine the external opening. It tracked directly inward. The fistula tracked subcutaneously then intersphincterically at the distal edge of the internal sphincter muscle. Hydrogen peroxide was injected, and the internal opening was identified. The fistula probe was then placed along the fistula tract. The overlying skin was incised to reveal subcutaneous tissue and the distal fibers of the internal sphincter muscle. A primary fistulotomy was then performed. Consideration had been given to placing the seton, however, the fistula track did not appear to involve the portion of the external sphincter muscle.

> Granulation tissue was present along the fistula tract. This was removed by curettage. The tract was inspected. There was no evidence of any side branches. The edges of the wound were then marsupialized to the fibrous base of the tract with two continuous 3-0 Vicryl sutures. The wound was irrigated and inspected. There was no evidence of any bleeding.

Assign the CPT procedure codes for the physician. _____

10. Rasjog P.

> **POSTOPERATIVE DIAGNOSIS:** Mild distal pouchitis.
> **PROCEDURE PERFORMED:** Ileoscopy of pelvic pouch.
> **PROCEDURE:** The patient was placed in the right lateral decubitus position and underwent an anal and perianal examination, which were unremarkable. The scope was then inserted into the patient's anal canal and from there easily into the pelvic pouch, which appeared to be easily distensible and pliable and found to contain a moderate amount of semi-formed fecal material. There was some diffuse erythema throughout the pouch, and in its distal portion there was evidence of fibrinous exudate. A biopsy was obtained and submitted for pathological examination. There was no active bleeding from the biopsy site. The anal canal was normal. The air was suctioned out and the scope withdrawn.

Assign the CPT procedure codes for the physician. _____

INTERNET RESEARCH

1. Visit Medicare's website to view coverage policies for virtual colonoscopy in your state: www.medicare.gov.
2. Visit the Human Anatomy Online website to learn more about the digestive system: www.innerbody.com/htm/body.html.
3. You can view procedures at the following website (free registration is required): http://or-live.com.
4. Learn more about digestive disorders at www.nlm.nih.gov/medlineplus/digestivesystem.html.

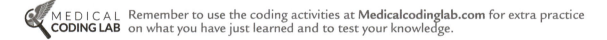 Remember to use the coding activities at **Medicalcodinglab.com** for extra practice on what you have just learned and to test your knowledge.

CPT: Urinary System

Chapter 22 in *Conquer Medical Coding* explains the correct coding and sequencing of diseases, injuries, and procedures included in the CPT's urinary system section. The organs covered by urology include the kidneys, ureters, urinary bladder, and urethra. Laparoscopic and cystourethroscopic procedures using an endoscope are common. The coder needs some knowledge of internal medicine, pediatrics, gynecology, and oncology to code correctly. The chapter also explains the following topics:

- The coding process used to assign correct codes for urethral dilation
- The three common methods of treating kidney stones via lithotripsy
- The purpose of urodynamic testing
- Open surgical procedures

CODE IT!

Supply the correct CPT codes required for the following cases.

1. _____ Cystourethroscopy with fulguration and excision of two large bladder tumors with steroid injection into the urethral stricture

2. _____ Endoscope used to pass through the urethra into the bladder and then the ureter; an electrohydraulic lithotriptor probe is used to pulverize the renal stone; an indwelling Double J stent is placed to facilitate passing of any residual stones

3. _____ Female patient has urethral stenosis; urologist performs a cystoscopy and internal urethrotomy with a 44 French urethrotome; cut was made at 11 o'clock; ureter orifices were in normal position

4. _____ Cystoscopy with urethral dilation and retrograde pyelogram of both ureters

5. _____ Kidney stone destroyed by directing shock waves through a liquid pad lying under the patient

6. _____ Litholapaxy of 3.0-cm bladder calculus

7. _____ An elderly woman presented to the emergency room with gross hematuria; acknowledges flank pain; a CT of the kidneys and ureters identified a mass of the right kidney; percutaneous needle biopsy of kidney is performed to rule out carcinoma

8. _____ CT examination of the abdomen; the CT images of the ureter demonstrate bilateral hydronephrosis and obstructing ureteral stones; cystourethroscopy with ureteroscopy and removal of right ureteral stones

9. _____ Surgical laparoscopy with ablation of renal cysts on the left

10. _____ Cystourethroscopy with insertion of Double J ureteral stent, right

MULTIPLE CHOICE

Select the option that best completes the statement or answers the question.

1. The surgeon removed a urinary calculus by making an incision directly into the kidney. What is this procedure called?
   A. Nephrectomy
   B. Nephrolithiasis
   C. Renal transection
   D. Nephrotomy

2. A female patient with chronic UTIs, hematuria, and frequency undergoes cystoscopy with biopsy of bladder outlet and incises the internal urethra. What is the correct way to code this situation?
   A. 52000, 52290
   B. 52204, 52270–51
   C. 52204, 52281–51
   D. 52204, 52276–51

3. A patient complains that he has the urge to urinate often yet when he goes, he doesn't void a large volume of urine despite straining to go. The physician performs a CMG with voiding pressure study and urethral pressure profile along with intra-abdominal voiding pressure study. What is the correct way to code this situation?
   A. 51727, 51728–51
   B. 51729, 51797
   C. 51726
   D. 51728, 51797

4. The physician performed a cystoscopy with fulguration of the bladder dome and removed calculus from the right ureter by inserting a urethroscope and catheter and grasping with stone basket forceps. What is the correct way to code this situation?
   A. 52214, 52352–51
   B. 52214, 52320–51
   C. 52224, 52310–51
   D. 52224, 52320–51

5. Which of the following measures how much urine the bladder can hold, how much pressure builds up inside the bladder as it stores urine, and the fullness at the urge to urinate?
   A. VP
   B. UPP
   C. EMG
   D. CMG

6. A patient is status post-prostate resection 5 years ago. He had a urinary sphincter placed for urinary incontinence and is now seen for removal and replacement of the device. What is the correct way to code this situation?
   A. 53442
   B. 53448
   C. 53449
   D. 53447

7. A patient has a renal calculus on the right. Lithotripsy is performed via cystoscopy with insertion of a Double J stent. What is the correct way to code this situation?
   A. 50980, 52332–RT–51
   B. 50561
   C. 52356
   D. 50575

8. A patient is found to have renal carcinoma. Previous surgeries were performed on this kidney over the years. The left kidney is removed via the open approach, leaving a partial ureter for hopes of future transplantation. What is the correct way to code this situation?
   A. 50225–LT
   B. 50220–LT
   C. 50234–LT
   D. 50546–LT

9. A patient with proteinuria, hematuria, diabetes, and chronic renal failure undergoes a percutaneous kidney biopsy on the right. What is the correct way to code this situation?
   A. 50020–RT
   B. 50200–RT
   C. 50045–RT
   D. 50574–RT

10. A 47-year-old female is experiencing loss of bladder control when jogging or squatting, and has increased frequency of urination. She is noted to have a hypermobile urethra. The physician performs an anterior urethropexy and sling for stress incontinence. What is the correct way to code this situation?
    A. 57288, 51820–51
    B. 51992, 51990–51
    C. 57288
    D. 51840, 57288–51

SHORT ANSWER

Answer the following questions.

1. A 63-year-old hypertensive female now has an enlarged kidney caused by blockage of the ureteral pelvic junction (UPJ). Her physician schedules a left renal endoscopy with ureteropy-elography, dilation of the ureter and UPJ, incision of the UPJ, and insertion of a stent through the renal pelvis into the UPJ. What are the correct code(s) and modifier, if applicable, for this procedure? _____

_____

2. A 68-year-old man presented with painless hematuria and urinary frequency. Cystoscopy demonstrates a circumferentially thickened bladder and a 1.0-cm eccentric mass along the posterior wall which was fulgurated. What are the correct code(s) and modifier, if applicable, for this procedure? _____

_____

3. A 69-year-old female with a 7-month history of stress incontinence is admitted for laparo-scopic urethral suspension. What are the correct code(s) and modifier, if applicable, for this procedure? _____

_____

4. The right renal allograft artery from a cadaver donor requires elongation before transplantation. A backbench arterial extension graft is performed. What are the correct code(s) and modifier, if applicable, for this procedure? _____

_____

5. A patient with post-void dribbling underwent a leak point pressure test along with an examination of the bladder through a cystourethroscopy approach. At the end of the procedure, the bladder was irrigated and all instruments removed. What are the correct code(s) and modifier, if applicable, for this procedure? _____

_____

6. This patient suffers from painful urination and blood in his urine. The urologist needs to examine both ureters and the bladder. She inserts a scope into the ureter(s), making an incision in the opening of the ureters to the bladder (meatotomy) and completes the examination. What are the correct code(s) and modifier, if applicable, for this procedure? _____

_____

7. A male patient complains of decreased urine output. On examination, he is experiencing suprapubic tenderness. He states he has only urinated twice in the last 24 hours. A 16-French Foley catheter was inserted to relieve the distended bladder and kidneys. What are the correct code(s) and modifier, if applicable, for this procedure? _____

_____

8. A patient is seen in the office complaining of feeling like she does not fully empty her bladder and has to make frequent trips to the bathroom. The physician performs a post-voiding residual ultrasound to measure how much urine remains in the bladder after voiding. What are the correct code(s) and modifier, if applicable, for this procedure? _____

_____

9. A male patient who is status post-prostatectomy is experiencing episodes of incontinence and complains that he feels like he is leaking urine throughout the day. He elects to proceed with a urethral sling to treat his incontinence in the outpatient surgery department. What are the correct code(s) and modifier, if applicable, for this procedure? _____

_____

10. A patient is seen after a 1-week bout with ureterolithiasis. The patient has not passed this stone as it is now lodged in the bladder. In the outpatient surgery center, the physician proceeds with cystoscopy with lithotripsy pulverization of a 2.5-cm stone. What are the correct code(s) and modifier, if applicable, for this procedure? _____

_____

CASE STUDIES

1. Arlo T.

> **OPERATION:** Meatotomy.
> **PROCEDURE:** After informed consent was obtained from the patient's mother, the patient was taken to the operating room and prepped and draped in the usual sterile manner in the supine position. The meatus was visualized and a straight hemostat used to crimp the urethral

meatus at the 6 o'clock position. Metzenbaum scissors were used to incise the crimped area. Redundant tissue was excised; 4-0 chromic was placed in an interrupted manner. Good hemostasis was noted. The urethral meatus was noted to be approximately an 8 French diameter at the conclusion of the meatotomy. Patient was stable when moved to the recovery room.

Assign the procedure code for the physician. _____

2. Collin D.

PROCEDURE PERFORMED: Flexible cystourethroscopy.
OPERATION: The patient was placed supine on the operating table and prepped and draped in sterile fashion. Intraurethral Xylocaine was instilled and, after an appropriate length of time, an Olympus flexible cystourethroscope was passed under direct vision. The anterior urethra was normal. The prostatic urethra was patent from the VERU. On cystoscopy there was grade 2 trabeculation with no evidence of tumors, ulcers, or calculi. The ureteral orifices were visualized with clear efflux bilaterally. The bladder neck was observed with no additional findings. The instrument was withdrawn and there were no additional findings. The patient tolerated the procedure well and left the operating room in satisfactory condition.

Assign the procedure code for the physician. _____

3. Mackie B.

PROCEDURE: Extracorporeal shock wave lithotripsy (ESWL).
INDICATIONS FOR OPERATION: The patient has had intermittent right renal colic. X-rays revealed a 9-mm calculus that was in the proximal ureter 2 weeks ago. The patient has continued to have some renal colic. He was scheduled for ESWL.
OPERATION: After fluoroscopy was performed and the stone was identified over the sacrum, the patient was induced and maintained on anesthesia and laryngeal mask airway (LMA). The stone was visualized in two planes and then subjected to 1,800 shocks. The intensity was raised to a maximum of 6 within the first 100 shocks and the patient tolerated this very well. No EKG changes. Frequency was left at 100 shocks per minute. At the end of 1,800 shocks, there was no calcific density remaining and the procedure was terminated. The patient was then awakened, extubated, and sent to the recovery room in good condition.

Assign the procedure code for the physician. _____

4. Grover M.

PROCEDURE: Cystoscopy with bladder biopsies and fulguration.
INDICATIONS: The patient is a 58-year-old male with a past history of superficial bladder cancer. Cystoscopy in the office recently has revealed irregular mucosa at the dome of his bladder. He now presents for bladder biopsies and fulguration.
OPERATION: A 21 French panendoscope was introduced into the bladder. At the right dome of the bladder, and along the right bladder wall, three separate areas were identified with irregular mucosa, each measuring 0.5 cm. Bladder biopsies were taken and these areas were fulgurated. The Bugbee electrode was used to cauterize all biopsy areas. The bladder was emptied and the scope removed. A 10-cc amount of 2% Xylocaine jelly was instilled per urethra.

Assign the procedure code for the physician. _____

5. Bethany S.

> **PREOPERATIVE DIAGNOSIS:** Carcinoma of the bladder.
> **OPERATION:** Resection of two bladder tumors.
> **PROCEDURE:** The patient was prepped and draped. The cystoscope was introduced and the bladder was examined. There was a large tumor mass arising in the posterior trigone on the left that extended onto the bladder wall. Resection was performed using coagulation and cauterization. A second tumor measuring 2.2 cm was located near the base of the larger resected tumor but had a different stalk. It was resected in toto. All chips were removed from the bladder. The base of the bladder was biopsied times two. Cauterization was carried out over the entire base. An 18 Foley catheter was placed.

Assign the procedure code for the physician. _____

6. Katrina J.

> **PROCEDURE DESCRIPTION:** Under satisfactory anesthesia, the patient was placed in the dorsolithotomy position. Using a #20 Wappler panendoscope sheath, right angle, and four oblique fiber-optic telescopes, a cystourethroscopy was performed with a normal urethra noted. The bladder was also unremarkable, but showed evidence of past reimplantation of the right ureter. Using a flexible ureteroscope, retrograde ureteroscopy was performed all the way to the renal pelvis. Two tumors were found in the upper ureter, one at the ureteropelvic junction and one below. Each was smaller than 0.5 cm in size. Using the rigid ureteroscope, the tumors were reached, and using a Bugbee electrode, fulguration of the tumors was carried out. Tissue that remained on the Bugbee was retained and sent to pathology for microscopic study. All of the instruments were removed, and the patient was moved to recovery in good condition.

Assign the procedure code for the physician. _____

7. Constance H.

> A patient with left ureteral stricture was admitted for treatment. As planned, cystourethroscopy with dilation of the left ureter stricture was performed and placement of indwelling stent was confirmed. The patient complained of right flank pain before the start of the case and the surgeon elected to perform a diagnostic cystourethroscopy with ureteroscopy of the right ureter.

Assign the procedure code for the physician. _____

8. Hector R.

> **PROCEDURE PERFORMED:** Extracorporeal shockwave lithotripsy; cystoscopy with Double J stent removal.
> The patient is a 59-year-old male who had undergone shockwave lithotripsy and ureteral stent placement previously for a partial staghorn calculus. The first lithotripsy fragmented approximately 40% of the stone, and he is presenting now to have the remainder of the stone treated.
> **OPERATION:** The patient was taken to the lithotripsy unit. He was placed on the lithotripsy table in a supine position. Following induction of anesthesia, fluoroscopy was used to position the patient where the stone was visualized in the focal point of the shockwaves. Shockwave lithotripsy was then performed. He was given a total of 4,000 shocks with a maximum power setting. Upon completion of the shocks, the patient was then transferred to the procedure room.
> The patient was then placed in the dorsal lithotomy position. The cystoscope was inserted through the urethra into the bladder. The Double J stent was located, grasped, and then extracted as the scope was pulled out.

Assign the procedure code for the physician. _____

9. Abrihoop S.

PROCEDURE: Closure of vesicostomy.

This boy was found to have a poorly compliant bladder with grade IV vesicoureteral reflux. A cutaneous vesicostomy was performed in 2000. The vesicoureteral reflux has not disappeared on the latest cystogram.

The patient was placed under general anesthesia and prepped and draped. The vesicostomy was circumscribed with the skin marking pencil and the scalpel. The incision was carried transversely on each side. Holding sutures of 3-0 silk were placed in the vesicostomy stoma. The fascia was freed by sharp scissor dissection circumferentially. The skin was freed. The bladder was freed by sharp scissor dissection from the fascia. The stoma was excised and the bladder was closed in three layers using one layer of running 2-0 chromic catgut, a layer of running 2-0 Vicryl, and a layer of interrupted 2-0 Vicryl. An 8 Dover Foley catheter was placed into the bladder with 3 cc in the balloon. The fascia was then closed with running suture of 2-0 Vicryl and reinforced with interrupted suture of 2-0 Vicryl. The skin was closed with running subcuticular suture 4-0 Monocryl. The Foley catheter was attached to a gravity drainage bag using the double diopter technique.

Assign the procedure code for the physician. _____

10. Samuel R.

The patient has a known ureteral stricture of the distal right ureter. Using ultrasound to guide the needle, it is placed through the skin and advanced into the distal portion of the right kidney. A glidewire is then advanced through this needle using fluoroscopy to guide it down the right ureter. The ureter is then dilated and an 8 French sheath is placed. A catheter is inserted and antegrade pyelogram is performed by injecting contrast to visualize the ureter and pelvis, showing a dilated ureter and renal pelvis. A stent is then placed.

Assign the procedure code for the physician. _____

INTERNET RESEARCH

1. Visit the OR-Live surgical archives website and view prerecorded urological procedures. Click on the procedure to see the video. You are required to register at no charge before the video is played. The video at www.or-live.com/hartfordhospital/1353 shows a procedure for urinary incontinence.
2. Search the Medicare coverage website for policies related to artificial sphincter procedures. Does Medicare cover this service? www.cms.gov/Center/Special-Topic/Medicare-Coverage-Center.html.
3. For more information on renal disorders, go to: www.renaldisorders.blogspot.com.

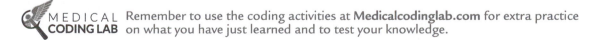 MEDICAL CODING LAB Remember to use the coding activities at **Medicalcodinglab.com** for extra practice on what you have just learned and to test your knowledge.

CPT: Male Genital System

Chapter 23 in *Conquer Medical Coding* explains the codes and terminology for the often-treated surgical cases involving the male genital system. The genitourinary system is the collective term used to describe all of the reproductive organs, as well as the organs responsible for creating and excreting urine. The genitourinary system can be affected by a wide range of clinical conditions, so knowledge of internal medicine, general surgery, and pediatrics is necessary. The chapter covers the following as well:

- The anatomical structures of the male genital system
- Newborn versus adult circumcision
- The techniques associated with hypospadias repair codes
- The various techniques for prostatectomy

CODE IT!

Assign all pertinent procedure codes, modifiers, and HCPCS codes.

1. _____ Orchiopexy in a 3-year-old boy for intra-abdominal testis

2. _____ Vasectomy in a 35-year-old

3. _____ Hydrocelectomy tunica vaginalis

4. _____ Revision of an incomplete circumcision

5. _____ Orchiectomy of the left testicle with insertion of prosthesis

6. _____ Needle biopsy of the prostate

7. _____ Cryosurgical ablation of the prostate

8. _____ Repeat transurethral resection of prostate tissue 4 years post original procedure

9. _____ Injection for Peyronie disease with exposure and injection of fibrous plaque

10. _____ Insertion of semi-rigid penile prosthesis

MULTIPLE CHOICE

Select the option that provides the correct code.

1. What is the correct way to code repair of a 2.0-cm laceration of the right testicle after a motorcycle accident?
   A. 12001
   B. 54670
   C. 54440
   D. 55899

2. What is the correct way to code an abdominal orchiopexy for left undescended testicle?
   A. 54560
   B. 54640
   C. 54692
   D. 54650

3. The urologist performs three needle biopsies of the prostate gland using ultrasonic guidance in the hospital. What is the correct way to code this situation?
   A. 55700 x3
   B. 55700 x3, 76942
   C. 55700, 76942–26
   D. 55700, 76942–51

4. A male patient presents with urinary retention, urethral stenosis, and vesical neck stenosis. The physician performs a meatotomy, urethral dilation, and a TURP. What is the correct way to code this situation?
   A. 52500, 53605–51
   B. 52601, 52510–51
   C. 52500, 52601
   D. 52601

5. The physician performs a biopsy of the right testis and performs a left radical orchiectomy-inguinal incision. What is the correct way to code this situation?
   A. 54530-LT
   B. 54530-LT, 54500-RT-51
   C. 54530-LT, 54500-RT-59
   D. 54530-LT, 54535

6. A patient with varicocele undergoes ligation of spermatic veins via endoscope. What is the correct way to code this situation?
   A. 55535
   B. 55550
   C. 55530
   D. 55559

7. The patient complains of multiple genital warts on the penis and scrotum. The physician applied trichloroacetic acid (TCA) to over 15 warts in several clusters. What is the correct way to code this situation?
   A. 54065
   B. 54056
   C. 54050
   D. 17004

8. The patient has a severe curvature of the penis. The physician incises the penis, exposing a 0.4-cm Peyronie plaque that is removed. What is the correct way to code this situation?
   A. 54205
   B. 11420
   C. 54110
   D. 11620

9. What is the correct way to code a MAGPI hypospadias repair with local skin flap during circumcision of a 2-year-old boy?
   A. 54332
   B. 54161
   C. 54322, 64161
   D. 54324

10. What is the correct way to code an excision lipoma of the right spermatic cord?
    A. 55520
    B. 55500
    C. 55520-RT
    D. 55550-RT

SHORT ANSWER

Answer the following questions.

1. A husband decides after remarrying that he wants to have more children and elects to have a vasectomy reversal performed bilaterally. Because this is such an intricate operation, the physician uses a microscope to reattach the vas deferens. What code(s) and modifier, if any, should be reported? _____

_____

2. A 4-year-old patient has had phimosis since birth with bleeding and pain. The patient was brought to the operating room for circumcision and was given a dorsal penile block with a modified ring block. What code(s) and modifier, if any, should be reported? _____

_____

3. A 40-year-old man has a 2-cm mass in the left scrotum. A frozen section is done intraoperatively, resulting in a diagnosis of benign adenoma tumor of the left scrotum. The tumor is excised. What code(s) and modifier, if any, should be reported? _____

_____

4. Diagnoses: Bilateral hydroceles; massive right spermatocele. Procedures: Bilateral hydrocelectomy with bottle procedure with right spermatocelectomy. What code should be reported? What code(s) and modifier, if any, should be reported? _____

_____

5. The patient is suffering from frequent urination, pressure, and pain in the bladder. Upon examination, the physician found dysplasia of the prostate. An incisional biopsy of the prostate was performed under local anesthesia to determine the nature of the dysplasia. What code(s) and modifier, if any, should be reported? _____

_____

6. A patient with a history of right testicular cancer found a lump on the left testicle during a monthly self-exam and feels his scrotum has slightly increased in size. The physician examined him and wants to rule out testicular tumor or spermatocele. The patient is seen in the outpatient surgery center for exploration of the scrotum and left testis. The physician performs a left inguinal exploration with spermatocelectomy and partial removal of the upper one-fourth epididymides. What code(s) and modifier, if any, should be reported? _____

_____

7. A patient presents to the office with complaints of a blister on his penis. This blister has been slowly increasing in size and is becoming irritated when it rubs against his clothing, inhibiting sexual activity. The physician examines his penis and diagnoses a boil. The physician incises the boil and applies antibiotic cream and a light dressing. What code(s) and modifier, if any, should be reported? _____

_____

8. A 9-year-old boy is seen in the ASC for orchiopexy for the right undescended testicle. When the scope entered the peritoneum, the surgeon discovered a small inguinal hernia sac in the right ilioinguinal canal and repaired this in addition to the orchiopexy on the right. What code should be reported? What code(s) and modifier, if any, should be reported? _____

_____

9. A 62-year-old male with prostate cancer undergoes elective prophylactic removal of the testes as part of his treatment with insertion of testicular prostheses. What code(s) and modifier, if any, should be reported? _____

_____

10. A male patient presents to the ED with abdominal pain and nausea for the last 10 hours. An ultrasound performed shows no evidence of appendicitis or intestinal blockage. Torsion of the left testicle is identified. The patient is admitted for surgical correction of the torsion and kept for observation. What code(s) and modifier, if any, should be reported? _____

_____

CASE STUDIES

1. Richard Y.

> **PREOPERATIVE DIAGNOSIS:** Phimosis.
> **POSTOPERATIVE DIAGNOSIS:** Phimosis.
> **PROCEDURE:** Circumcision.
> **PROCEDURE IN DETAIL:** After the induction of general anesthesia, this 24-year-old patient was prepped and draped in the supine position. A straight hemostat was placed on the dorsal surface of the foreskin and left in place for 15 seconds. This was removed, and scissors were used to cut along this line. A straight hemostat was placed on the ventral surface of the foreskin and left in place for 15 seconds. Scissors were used to cut along this line. The excess foreskin was excised in freehand fashion using curved scissors. Bleeding points were coagulated with electrocautery. The foreskin was re-approximated using interrupted sutures of 3-0 chromic. 0.5% Marcaine was then injected for post-op local anesthesia. Vaseline and 4 × 4 dressings were applied.

Assign the code(s) and modifier for the physician. _____

2. Andrew T.

> **PREOPERATIVE DIAGNOSIS:** Left spermatocele.
> **OPERATIVE PROCEDURE:** Left spermatocelectomy.
> **DESCRIPTION OF SURGERY:** The patient was taken to the operating suite and positioned in the supine position with the shaved scrotum exposed. A midline incision was made and taken down to the dartos layer. The large multiloculated spermatocele was identified. It was approximately 6 cm in greatest diameter. We got down to the avascular layer, and dissected free and

circumferentially down to its base arising from the upper end of the epididymis. At this point, it was cross-clamped and dissected, thus removing the structure. I oversewed the stump with #3-0 Vicryl. Hemostasis was meticulously secured. The testicle was replaced within the right hemiscrotum. The dartos layer was closed with #3-0 Vicryl. The skin was closed with #4-0 chromic in a horizontal, interrupted fashion. OPSITE spray dressing was applied. Scrotal support was placed over a fluffed gauze dressing.

Assign the code(s) and modifier for the physician. _____

3. Niguel S.

PREOPERATIVE DIAGNOSIS: Hypospadias.
OPERATIVE PROCEDURE: Repair of hypospadias (Snodgrass procedure).
SUMMARY: The patient is a 10-month-old baby boy with the previously mentioned anomaly admitted for repair.
DESCRIPTION OF SURGERY: The patient's penis was noted with subcoronal hypospadias. There was no significant chordee. The penis was completely degloved to increase its overall length. The urethra was reconstructed through the subcoronal area to the tip of the penis using Snodgrass, incised, tubularized, urethral plate. The procedure was done in two layers of #7-0 PDS. The glans penis was closed on top of the reconstructed urethra with two layers of #7-0 PDS as well. Redundant foreskin was removed. Circumcision and midline incisions were closed with running interrupted #6-0 chromic sutures. Dermabond glue and a Tegaderm dressing were applied. The patient left the operating room in good condition. There were no complications or blood loss.

Assign the code(s) and modifier for the physician. _____

4. Brian O.

PREOPERATIVE DIAGNOSIS: Chordee.
OPERATION: Repair of chordee.
The patient is a 12-month-old baby boy with congenital chordee admitted for repair.
PROCEDURE: The patient was brought to the operating room, identified, prepped and draped in the usual sterile manner, and placed in the supine position under general anesthesia. Exam under anesthesia revealed a 90-degree chordee with a ventral bend. A circumferential incision was performed and the penis was completely degloved, resecting the whole chordee tissue. An artificial erection was performed which confirmed a completely straight penis. The foreskin was rearranged to accommodate a longer ventral surface. Circumcision and midline incisions were closed with running #6-0 chromic sutures. A Tegaderm dressing was applied. The patient left the operating room in good condition. There were no complications or blood loss.

Assign the code(s) and modifier for the physician. _____

5. Gabriel L.

PREOPERATIVE DIAGNOSIS: Redundant foreskin with phimosis.
OPERATION: Revision for incomplete circumcision in 10-year-old boy.
ANESTHESIA: General with dorsal penile block.
PROCEDURE: Examination of the phallus revealed significant redundant foreskin covering almost the entire glans. The meatus was normal. There was no chordee. At this point I administered a dorsal penile block with 0.25% Marcaine without epinephrine. I then made a proximal circumferential skin incision at the level of the coronal impression. A second circumferential skin incision was made distally, leaving a rim of mucosa with a glans of about 45 mm. The foreskin was incised dorsally and then resected from the shaft sharply. Hemostasis was secured with

careful electrocautery. The skin edges were then re-approximated with interrupted sutures of #5-0 chromic. The final cosmetic result was excellent. Hemostasis was excellent. The child had received Ancef 250 mg IV preoperatively. A sterile dressing was applied.

Assign the code(s) and modifier for the physician. _____

6. Scott J.

PREOPERATIVE DIAGNOSIS: Abnormal PSA.
PROCEDURE: Transrectal ultrasound of the prostate and ultrasound-guided prostate biopsies.
INDICATIONS: This is a 68-year-old man with an abnormal PSA of 6.3. His prostate gland is enlarged but smooth.
OPERATION: Prostate ultrasound images were obtained in the transverse and longitudinal planes. Total gland volume was 107 cc with a gland length of 64.8 mm. The prostate capsule appears intact. The seminal vesicles are enlarged but symmetric. In the central gland, a large amount of hypertrophy is noted. In the peripheral zone, several small hypoechoic areas are seen. After injection of 10 cc of 1% lidocaine through a spinal needle to the angle of seminal vesicles, six biopsies were taken from each lobe of the prostate. The patient tolerated the procedure well and was returned to the dressing area in stable condition.
PATHOLOGY REPORT: All biopsies were consistent with benign prostatic hyperplasia.

Assign the code(s) and modifier for the physician. _____

7. Hu C.

PREOPERATIVE DIAGNOSIS: Elective sterilization.
PROCEDURE PERFORMED: Bilateral vasectomy.
OPERATION: In the physician office, the patient was placed in the supine position on the procedure table, where he was shaved, prepped, and draped in a sterile fashion. Using 2% local Xylocaine, the left vas was isolated with towel clips. Sharp and blunt dissection was then used to deliver a 2.5-cm portion of the left vas, which was clamped and excised. Hemostasis was achieved with electrocautery. The vasal lumen were then electrofulgurated and the stumps were ligated with 3-0 chromic catgut suture. In addition, the fascia was oversewn with 3-0 chromic catgut. Having achieved satisfactory hemostasis, the vasal stumps were replaced in the scrotal sac. The primary skin incision was closed with interrupted 3-0 plain catgut sutures. A similar procedure was carried out, uneventfully, on the right side. Betadine ointment, together with gauze and a scrotal support, were applied to the operative site. The patient was given instructions regarding postoperative care and the need to maintain contraception until a negative semen specimen was obtained. He otherwise tolerated the procedure well and left the operating room in satisfactory condition.

Assign the code(s) and modifier for the physician. _____

8. Durward E.

PREOPERATIVE DIAGNOSIS: Abdominal left testis.
PROCEDURE: Second-stage laparoscopic-assisted right orchidopexy on vas.
This boy was found to have a nonpalpable right undescended testis. He previously underwent laparoscopy wherein the first stage of the procedure was performed when spermatic vessels were clipped with 5-mm clips. He is here today for stage II. An 8 French pediatric ceding tube was inserted into the bladder and placed on sterile gravity drainage during the procedure. Punctures were made at the umbilicus and the anterior superior iliac spine. The right testis was noted in the abdominal location and peeping into the internal ring. The spermatic vessels were identified and the clip was seen. The spermatic vessels were then freed laterally. The peritoneum was freed proximally using the scissor and the coagulating current on 15. The testicle

was then freed from its attachments to the internal ring. This was done laterally. Using the grasping forceps and a dissector, alternately, the gubernaculums were pulled into the abdomen. The testicle now seemed to have adequate length to reach into the scrotum. Accordingly, a small transverse incision was made in the lower portion of the scrotum. Two sutures were placed in the lower level of the scrotum. A Schnidt clamp was then passed through the scrotal incision and into the abdomen lateral to the bladder but medial to the inferior epigastric vessels. The opening was dilated and the Schnidt clamp was used to grasp the testis, which was pulled down to the scrotum. The testicle was anchored in place with the two sutures of 3-0 Vicryl. Trocars were removed after removing the carbon dioxide. There were no complications.

Assign the code(s) and modifier for the physician. _____

9. Billy Joe F.

PATIENT STATUS: Post-prostatectomy complaints of impotence.
Billy Joe has a problematic complication affecting many males after a prostatectomy. He has tried several prescription medications for impotence with limited success. Billy Joe elects to have a semirigid penile prosthesis inserted. The physician makes a transverse incision on the penis above the pubic bone. Dissection is carried down at the base of the penis to the erectile tissues, making sure to avoid nerves and blood vessels. The incision is carried down into the corpora cavernosa. Dilators are inserted one at a time down each side of the penis. Prostheses are then inserted down the length of the penile shaft. Incisions are closed.

Assign the code(s) and modifier (if any) for the physician. _____

10. Georgios P.

PREOPERATIVE DIAGNOSES: Undescended right testis.
PROCEDURE: Laparoscopy; redo right orchidopexy.
The patient had a right hernia repair and orchidopexy at age 1 year and 6 months. The testis is no longer in position. The patient is placed under general anesthesia and a Foley catheter is placed. The abdomen is filled with CO_2 using the Veress needle. A trocar is inserted and inspection of the abdomen showed on the right that the vas and vessels were going to the internal ring and scar tissue was present from the previous surgery. On the left, exploration was carried out; the vas and vessels seemed to end blindly and did not connect with the internal ring. A second puncture was made in the abdomen anterior to the iliac crest and a 5-mm probe was passed to free the sigmoid colon. The left testis is not present. CO_2 was removed and the skin was closed with stitches.
A large oblique right groin incision was made as the testis was palpable in the groin. The testis was freed from its attachments. The scar tissue extended all the way to the internal ring. This was freed millimeter by millimeter. The vas was freed and the lateral spermatic ligaments were freed. The peritoneal reflexion was freed by sharp dissection. The testis now had enough length to reach down to the scrotum. The testis was then anchored within the scrotum. The inguinal canal was closed, followed by the external oblique aponeurosis. Foley catheter is removed.

a. *Is the urinary catheterization coded separately?* _____

b. *Assign the code(s) and modifier for the physician.* _____

INTERNET RESEARCH

1. Visit www.thedoctorschannel.com/channels/urology and review some of the latest news in urology and treating male genital conditions. Research a topic that is of particular interest to you.
2. Visit http://uro.broadcastmed.com and watch various prostate surgeries and read up on robotic prostate surgeries.

MEDICAL CODING LAB   Remember to use the coding activities at **Medicalcodinglab.com** for extra practice on what you have just learned and to test your knowledge.

CPT: Female Genital System and Maternity Care and Delivery

Chapter 24 in *Conquer Medical Coding* explains the procedural coding and terminology of the most common diseases, disorders, and surgical treatment of the female genital and reproductive systems. The genitourinary system is the collective term used to describe all of the reproductive organs and the organs responsible for creating and excreting urine. Coders should be aware that many procedures are able to be performed in more than one way. Correct code assignment requires determining the approach that is documented. The female genital section of the CPT is arranged by anatomical site and then by type of root procedure. The chapter explains the following topics as well:

- The difference among laparoscopic, hysteroscopic, colposcopic, and open surgical procedures
- The procedures that are provided as part of an annual examination
- The appropriate hysterectomy procedure code based on seven criteria
- The services inclusive in the maternity and delivery global package
- The differences between elective and therapeutic abortions and the various techniques
- The assisted reproductive technology treatments for infertility

CODE IT!

Supply the correct codes for the following.

1. _____ Patient with CIN II who undergoes conization of the cervix with LEEP

2. _____ Excision of Bartholin's gland abscess

3. _____ Laparoscopic fimbrioplasty

4. _____ Laparoscopic chromotubation of the oviducts to rule out obstruction of both fallopian tubes in patient who has been unable to conceive

5. _____ Procedure: D&C for incomplete miscarriage. Diagnosis: Spontaneous miscarriage, 21 weeks, incomplete.

6. _____ Cervical cerclage via vaginal approach for a 27-year-old female, 19 weeks' gestation, who presents with an incompetent cervix

7. _____ Laparotomy with removal of four subserosal leiomyomata

8. _____ Patient with hematometrium and cervical stenosis undergoes cervical dilation with release of retained blood followed by endometrial curettage with ultrasound guidance.

9. _____ An anterior colporrhaphy performed on a 55-year-old patient to correct a vaginal cystocele

10. _____ A 68-year-old female is seen for her annual GYN exam. Pelvic and clinical breast exam are performed in addition to cervical and vaginal cancer screening

MULTIPLE CHOICE

Select the option that provides the correct code.

1. A hysteroscopy was performed with biopsy of the endometrium and D&C. What is the correct way to code this situation?
   A. 58558, 58120–51
   B. 58558
   C. 58100, 58120–51
   D. 58558–52

2. Code(s) for colposcopy, cervical biopsy, and endocervical curettage performed at the same setting.
   A. 57454
   B. 57421
   C. 57455, 57456
   D. 57456

3. A patient has a D&C on Tuesday; findings indicate the necessity for a TAH, which is performed the following week. What is the correct way to code this situation?
   A. 57800, 58150
   B. 57800, 58150–51
   C. 58120, 58150–58
   D. 58120, 76942–51

4. A patient presents with vesicouterine fistula—the physician performs a closure of the fistula. What is the correct way to code this situation?
   A. 51920
   B. 51900
   C. 51925
   D. 51900–22

5. A patient has a malignant pelvic mass. The physician performs an exploratory laparotomy, bilateral salpingo-oopherectomy, omental biopsy, omentectomy, and pelvic washings. What is the correct way to code this situation?
   A. 58953
   B. 58950
   C. 58960
   D. 58950, 58900–59

6. A female patient presents with cystocele and rectocele. The physician performs an anteroposterior colporrhaphy to repair the defect. What is the correct way to code this situation?
   A. 57240, 57250–59
   B. 57260, 57240–59
   C. 57260
   D. 57240, 57250–51

7. An obstetrician performs a total abdominal hysterectomy immediately following a cesarean section delivery due to the patient's badly damaged uterus. Code for the procedure(s) and routine antepartum and postpartum care.
   A. 59510, 59525
   B. 59510, 59525–51
   C. 59610, 59525
   D. 59610, 59525–59

8. The physician delivers twins on Tuesday. While still in the hospital, the patient had a tubal ligation performed. Code for the tubal ligation.
   A. 58600
   B. 58605
   C. 58605–50
   D. 58600–50

9. A patient has a vaginal delivery after a previous cesarean delivery; the physician provided antepartum and postpartum care. What is the correct way to code this situation?
   A. 59610, 59614–51
   B. 59610
   C. 59610–22, 59614–51
   D. 59610–22

10. A patient is admitted for repair of an enterocele. The physician performs a McCall culdoplasty via abdominal approach with mesh. What is the correct way to code this situation?
    A. 57265, 57267
    B. 57270, 57267
    C. 57268
    D. 57270

SHORT ANSWER

Answer the following questions.

1. Because of the patient's long-term excessive vaginal bleeding, a D&C was performed post vaginal delivery. What code(s) will be reported? _____

\
_____

2. An on-call OB physician delivers a child for a patient assigned to her from the ED. The patient received intermittent prenatal care at the health department. The baby was not progressing, necessitating an episiotomy and external cephalic version. The OB physician plans to see the patient for follow up in 6 weeks. What code(s) will be reported? _____

\
_____

3. A 70-year-old patient is diagnosed with vaginal carcinoma. She had her ovaries removed 5 years ago for an ovarian mass that was diagnosed as uncertain pathology. She now presents for vaginectomy, complete removal of vaginal wall. What code(s) will be reported? _____

\
_____

4. A patient in her 23rd week of pregnancy underwent amniocentesis because of her advanced maternal age and low APR test. After being counseled about the chromosomal abnormality of her fetus, she elects to have a therapeutic abortion. D&C is performed under general anesthesia. What code(s) will be reported? _____

\
_____

5. The patient suffers from vaginal intraepithelial neoplasia. The vagina and vaginal cuff were sprayed with vinegar solution, after which white epithelium appeared. Areas were injected with Marcaine, after which the area was completely vaporized with a CO_2 laser. The area vaporized was the size of a silver dollar. What code(s) will be reported? _____

6. A patient with severe introital dyspareunia and chronic inflammation of the perineum and vestibule undergoes vulvar vestibulectomy with perineoplasty. The posterior perineal and vestibular abnormal and inflamed-looking tissue was marked with a surgical pen and excised beyond 7 cm. What code(s) will be reported? _____

7. Patient is gravida 6, para 3, and admitted at 38 weeks' gestation and is fully dilated. The physician has followed this patient for the length of her pregnancy. She has a +3 station with moderate meconium staining of fluid. The physician performs amnioinfusion during labor with good results and notes moderate clearing of the amniotic fluid. With epidural anesthesia, the patient delivers by spontaneous vaginal delivery. Assign the code reported by the anesthesiologist. _____ Assign the code for the OB/GYN. _____

8. A 37-year-old pregnant patient has been bleeding for 4 days. She is diagnosed with a spontaneous incomplete miscarriage at 15 weeks. She is treated in the outpatient surgery center with D&C. This is her fourth miscarriage due to incompetent cervix. What code(s) will be reported? _____

9. A 15-year-old patient is admitted for induction of labor at 39 weeks 5/7 days because of decreased fetal movement. The patient is induced with Pitocin drip and becomes fully dilated. She is unable to push because of exhaustion and the epidural. The physician performs a low vacuum outlet extraction delivery using a Mityvac vacuum with three pulls, and then performs an episiotomy. What code(s) will be reported? _____

10. A patient is admitted for a scheduled repeat low segment transverse cesarean section. The patient, who is term at 39 weeks, also signs a consent form for sterilization at the time of her C-section. A 7 pound 15 ounce girl is delivered and tubal ligation is carried out immediately after suturing the uterus. What code(s) will be reported? _____

CASE STUDIES

1. Crissy H.

> **PROCEDURE:** Diagnostic hysteroscopy with D&C.
> A pelvic exam was performed. A weighted speculum was placed, and single tooth tenaculum was placed anteriorly on the cervix. A diagnostic hysteroscope was introduced into the endocervix on direct visualization and into the intrauterine cavity. This was withdrawn and the cervix dilated to #8 Hagar. A sharp uterine curette was introduced and the uterine cavity was systematically curetted with a minimal amount of tissue.

Assign the procedure code for the physician. _____

2. Jaidyn N.

PREOPERATIVE DIAGNOSIS: Multiparity; desires sterility.
OPERATION: Laparoscopic bilateral tubal ligation.
PROCEDURE: The urinary bladder was drained and a uterine manipulator was placed. A small infraumbilical incision was created with the scalpel blade. The step trocar was inserted without difficulty. A pneumoperitoneum was created once proper placement was confirmed.
The camera was inserted and detailed visual examination was carried out. A suprapubic trocar was inserted under direct visualization with care taken to avoid injuring the intra-abdominal contents. The right fallopian tube was traced to its fimbriated end and a Falope ring was applied to the isthmic portion of the tube. Proper placement was confirmed. A similar procedure was carried out on the opposite side. Proper placement of both Falope rings was confirmed visually.

Assign the procedure code for the physician. _____

3. Darlene O.

PREOPERATIVE DIAGNOSIS: Cervical dysplasia with atypia.
OPERATION: Laser ablation of the cervix.
PROCEDURE: The perineum was prepped, and a speculum was inserted into the vagina. A 3% ascetic acid was placed on the cervix. An area of dysplasia was noted 0.5 cm around the cervical os. Next, 14 cc of 1 amp Pitressin and 50 cc of normal saline were injected into the cervix. The area was ablated 7 cm deep using a CO_2 laser at 40 watts. The rest of the cervix was brushed using a 20-watt laser. Good hemostasis was noted and the speculum was removed.

Assign the procedure code for the physician. _____

4. Lilyana C.

POSTOPERATIVE DIAGNOSIS:
1. Dysmenorrhea
2. Menorrhagia
3. Mild pelvic endometriosis
OPERATION:
1. Diagnostic laparoscopy
2. Fulguration of endometriosis
3. Hysteroscopy
4. D&C (dilation and curettage)
5. Ablation
PROCEDURE: After good general anesthesia, a speculum was placed in the vagina and the anterior lip of the cervix was grasped. The cervical os was dilated and a Kohn's cannula was placed in the os. A Foley catheter was inserted to drain the bladder. The infraumbilical area and suprapubic area were infiltrated with Marcaine with epinephrine and a stab wound was made at the umbilicus.
A Veress needle was inserted through the step trocar sheath; the abdomen was insufflated and the trocar placed through the sheath. It entered the abdomen without evidence of damage. A second puncture was performed two finger breadths from the symphysis pubis. The uterus was slightly enlarged but otherwise appeared normal. There were white lesions consistent with endometriosis in the cul de sac. One dark lesion was apparent on the right distal fallopian tube. These areas were fulgurated with the bipolar. A simple cyst in the left ovary was drained with the bipolar with good hemostasis noted.
Her legs were repositioned and the weighted speculum placed in the vagina. The anterior lip of the cervix had been grasped and the hysteroscope was inserted. The cavity was normal appearing. Sharp and suction curettage was performed. The ThermaChoice balloon was placed

and pressure was stabilized at 175 mm Hg; an 8-minute therapy cycle was run without difficulty. The balloon was removed, after which the instruments and gas were removed from above. The incisions were closed with 4-0 Vicryl subcuticular stitches.

a. *A D&C was actually performed: True or false?* _____

b. *The diagnostic laparoscopy is reported separately: True or false?* _____

c. *Assign the procedure code for the physician.* _____

5. Silvia A.

> **POSTOPERATIVE DIAGNOSIS:** Fibroepithelial vaginal polyp.
> **OPERATION:** Excision of fibroepithelial polyp.
> The patient has a 2- to 3-cm prolapsing polyp from the anterior aspect of her vagina, which is troublesome and in the way. She is requesting excision.
> **OPERATIVE FINDINGS:** Examination under anesthesia revealed a 3-cm vaginal polyp, prolapsing out the vagina, attached at 1:00. Using cautery set at 70/30 and a large loop attachment, the polyp was excised. Cautery was performed of the base, and a few sutures were used.
> **OPERATIVE SUMMARY AND TECHNIQUES:** Before removal, about 1 cc of Marcaine without epinephrine was injected around the base of the polyp. Using a large, flat loop attached to cautery set at 70/30 cut/coag, the polyp was removed in one fell swoop. The base of the polyp was then cauterized with a ball cautery set at 50/50. Three sutures of 2.0 chromic were then placed to re-approximate the edges for further hemostasis.

Assign the procedure code for the physician. _____

6. Thanh T.

> **PREOPERATIVE and POSTOPERATIVE DIAGNOSIS:** Failed intrauterine pregnancy, 11 weeks.
> **OPERATION:** D&C.
> **PROCEDURE:** The patient was taken to the operating room in the supine position. Anesthesia was instituted and the patient was prepped and draped in the dorsal lithotomy position. The bladder was drained and the cervix isolated. The uterus was sounded and the cervix was dilated to accommodate an 8-mm suction curette. Tissue and blood were removed. Sharp curettage was performed, and the suction curette was used once again to remove the remaining clots of blood. Sharp curette was once again performed to ensure adequacy of procedure. Good hemostasis was noted.

Assign the procedure code for the physician. _____

7. Savannah I.

> **POSTOPERATIVE DIAGNOSIS:** Menorrhagia, dysfunctional uterine bleeding.
> **PROCEDURE PERFORMED:**
> 1. Hysteroscopy
> 2. Dilatation and curettage
> 3. Myomectomy
> 4. Paracervical block
> **DESCRIPTION OF PROCEDURE:** The cervix was visualized and a paracervical block was performed using a total of 10 cc of 1% lidocaine plain, which was injected at 12, 3, 6, and 9 o'clock on the cervix. The patient tolerated that procedure well. Sequential Hegar dilators were used to dilate the internal cervical os. Before that, the uterine sound had been used to define the length of the endometrial cavity, which was found to be 12 cm in length. The right side of the endometrial cavity was found to be irregular in contour, consistent with bulky fibroids involving the right half of the uterine fundus. The cavity itself was thus distorted slightly to the left and was slightly retroverted in its orientation. The hysteroscope was introduced and both cornua were

visualized without problems. The endometrial lining was found to be pale and hemorrhagic with a great deal of blood as the patient was at the end of her menses. The hysteroscope was then removed and curettage was performed in all quadrants until a gritty texture was noted. The endometrial curettings were sent to pathology. At this point, the scope was reinserted and a large 3-cm anterior fibroid was removed. Following that, all instruments were removed from the vagina.

Assign the procedure code for the physician. _____

8. Kellyn M.

Kellyn, who has a high-risk pregnancy, is carrying twins. At 32 weeks, she presents to the hospital in labor. She delivers the first baby vaginally. The second baby is in the transverse lie position requiring C-section.

What codes will the obstetrician report? a. Baby 1: _____ *b. Baby 2:* _____

9. Jia T.

PREOPERATIVE DIAGNOSIS: Patient desires permanent sterilization.
OPERATION: Laparoscopic tubal ligation by cautery and transection.
PROCEDURE: A weighted speculum was placed into the vagina. A tenaculum was placed on the anterior lip of the cervix. The cervix was grasped gently and attached to a suction cannula; then, the tenaculum was removed. A vertical subumbilical incision was made with a knife and the Veress needle was gently placed intraperitoneally. Opening pressure was 4 mm Hg. The abdomen was insufflated with approximately 2.5 liters of carbon dioxide. The Ethicon disposable trocar was inserted with the first attempt. The suprapubic 5-mm port was placed in the standard fashion with the Ethicon disposable cannula without difficulty. The Kleppinger forceps were placed through the suprapubic incision, and the right fallopian tube was grasped in its mid portion and carefully visualized and photographed. The fimbriae were visualized and then cauterized four times with excellent blanching effect. They were then transected with the Bock scissors. The same procedure was carried out on the left side. There was no evidence of adhesions. The intestines appeared normal. The gas was allowed to egress and the instruments were removed under direct visualization. The incisions were closed with 4-0 Vicryl.

Assign the procedure code for the physician. _____

10. Sheila R.

PREOPERATIVE and POSTOPERATIVE DIAGNOSIS:
1. Pelvic pain
2. Dyspareunia
OPERATION: Revision of hymen.
INDICATIONS: Patient is a pleasant 22-year-old female with persistent dyspareunia limited to the posterior hymen. Patient has a narrow vaginal outlet.
PROCEDURE: Allis clamps were placed on the posterior fourchette and the posterior hymen was incised in a vertical fashion. A small portion of vaginal tissue was excised and sent to pathology for evaluation. The incision was re-approximated in a horizontal fashion using interrupted 2-0 chromic suture. Hemostasis was confirmed.

Assign the procedure code for the physician. _____

INTERNET RESEARCH

1. Visit www.acog.org. Select *Practice Management* and then *Coding*. Read any frequently asked questions or articles about reporting E/M codes or the global obstetrics code when a patient is seen to confirm a pregnancy test. What do they say about this? When can the E/M be reported?
2. Visit Aetna's website at www.aetna.com and search for "endometrial ablation" to locate the clinical policy for this procedure. What criteria must be met before the insurer will authorize endometrial ablation?

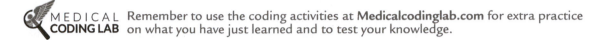 Remember to use the coding activities at **Medicalcodinglab.com** for extra practice on what you have just learned and to test your knowledge.

CPT: Endocrine and Nervous Systems

Chapter 25 in *Conquer Medical Coding* explains the procedural coding and terminology for surgical treatment of the central nervous system and endocrine system as outlined in the CPT. The endocrine system section represents codes for glands that release their hormones directly into the bloodstream. The nervous system section covers many procedures on the skull, meninges, brain, spine, spinal cord, and nerves. Some of the procedures in this section are accomplished endoscopically; however, most of them are carried out by open technique. This chapter also explains the following topics:

- The anatomical structures of the endocrine and nervous systems
- The common treatments of nerve pain: neurolysis, neuroplasty, neurorrhaphy, and nerve blocks
- When it is appropriate to report nerve blocks separately from the anesthesia provided for the surgery
- The various methods of nerve repair: nerve graft, nerve wrapping, and suture repair
- The purpose of neurostimulators and their components
- When procedure codes from both the musculoskeletal and nervous system sections are required when reporting services performed on the spine
- The purpose of the common spinal procedures: discectomy, decompression, corpectomy, and laminectomy

CODE IT!

Supply the correct codes for the following.

1. _____ Obese patient seeking treatment for excessive hunger who receives intra-abdominal avulsion of the vagus nerve

2. _____ Two ulnar nerves microscopically sutured in the hand in the ED after an electric saw accident

3. _____ Patient suffering from debilitating back pain for over a year who is admitted for percutaneous epidural implantation of neurostimulator and four electrodes

4. _____ Excision of thyroid adenoma

5. _____ Implantation of a ventricular catheter through a burr hole by a neurosurgeon

6. _____ Craniectomy performed to excise a meningioma in the posterior fossa

7. _____ A thyroid lobe, freed from its attachments to the adjacent structures, which is then completely freed by cutting through the isthmus and detaching it from the trachea

8. _____ Surgery of a 15-mm aneurysm, intracranial approach, carotid circulation

9. _____ Biopsy of trigeminal nerve

10. _____ Patient who suffers from pseudotumor cerebri undergoes a lumbar puncture to lessen the CSF pressure

MULTIPLE CHOICE

Select the option that best provides the correct code, completes the statement, or answers the question.

1. The adrenal glands are:
   A. At the base of the brain
   B. In the mediastinum of the chest
   C. On top of each kidney
   D. Just below each skin layer

2. How should you code the excision of an adenoma from the posterior aspect of the thyroid gland?
   A. 60100
   B. 60200
   C. 60200–22
   D. 60210

3. How should you code for partial excision of both lobes of the thyroid with removal of the isthmus?
   A. 60210
   B. 60210, 60212
   C. 60225
   D. 60212

4. A patient has a resection of neoplasm, midline skull base, extradural, using the infratemporal preauricular approach to the middle cranial fossa. The otolaryngologist performed the approach, whereas the neurosurgeon performed the definitive procedure. Provide each code that would be billed by each surgeon.
   A. 61590, 61607
   B. 61591, 61607
   C. 61590, 61607–51
   D. 61518

5. How should you code the removal of a complete cerebrospinal fluid shunt system, with replacement?
   A. 62256
   B. 62258
   C. 62256, 62258
   D. 62256, 62258–51

6. The patient has right trigeminal neuralgia, and Gamma knife stereotactic surgery is performed. The head frame was placed prior to the procedure. What is the correct way to code this situation?
   A. 61796, 61795
   B. 61796
   C. 64600, 61795
   D. 61795

7. The patient is admitted with a diagnosis of cerebral aneurysm. The surgeon performs an intracranial aneurysm repair by intracranial approach with microdissection, carotid circulation. What is the correct way to code this situation?
   A. 61700
   B. 61700, 69990–51
   C. 61700, 69990
   D. 61703, 69990

8. A patient has persistent pain of the low back and leg subsequent to an MVA 5 years ago. The sacral area is prepped and a needle is placed in the caudal space, administering Xylocaine and Decadron to block the pain. What is the correct way to code this situation?
   A. 62323
   B. 62326
   C. 62323, 77003–26
   D. 62326, 77003–26

9. A neurosurgeon performs implantation of a ventricular catheter through a burr hole. What is the correct way to code this situation?
   A. 61020
   B. 61105
   C. 61210
   D. 61107

10. A patient is suffering from intracranial hemorrhage resulting from an intracranial aneurysm in the right carotid artery. Emergent microdissection of the aneurysm via intracranial approach is performed. What is the correct way to code this situation?
    A. 61700, 69990
    B. 61700
    C. 61697
    D. 61697, 69990

SHORT ANSWER

Answer the following questions.

1. A patient suffering from general weakness and dizziness is sent for a CT scan. The scan reveals a supratentorial brain abscess that must be excised. A craniectomy, trephination, and bone flap craniotomy are performed and the abscess is excised. What code(s) will be reported? _____

   _____

2. A patient with kidney cancer had his left kidney and left adrenal gland removed. Based on CPT coding guidelines, can the surgeon report the kidney removal code and code 60540? (Carefully review code 60540 for an important CPT concept in surgical coding.) Explain your answer. _____

   _____

   _____

   _____

3. The physician documented partial midline C3–C4 corpectomies with removal of 40% of the vertebra and discectomy. Should the doctor report code 63081 or 63075? Explain your answer. _____

   _____

   _____

   _____

4. A patient with thoracic radiculopathy and a herniated disk is being treated with percutaneous discectomy at T4–T5. A C-arm is used for fluoroscopic guidance. The physician inserts a spinal needle and injects local anesthetic. A 17-gauge introducer needle is then inserted into the disk. The physician inserts a spine-wand and several passes are made into the disk; radiofrequency vaporization and coagulation are then carried out for 8 seconds at each pass. At the end of the procedure, the disk space is collapsed with decompression accomplished. Assign the codes for this service. _____

   _____

   _____

5. A long-time pain clinic patient has failed all conservative treatments as well as injections. He is seen today for placement of intracranial neurostimulator electrodes in the cortex via burr holes for long-term pain relief. Assign the codes for this service. _____

   _____

6. A patient has had difficulty walking with associated hand pain on the same side. An MRI shows spondylolisthesis at C5–C6. Anterior discectomy is performed with decompression of the spinal cord and osteophytectomy in the interspace of C5 and C6. Assign the codes for this service. _____

   _____

7. A patient suffering from radiculitis caused by a herniated disk and nucleus pulposus and spinal stenosis is admitted to observation following a laminectomy, decompression of the spinal nerve root L2–L3 with partial resection of the facet bone, and foraminotomy.

   a. What region was the procedure performed on? _____

   b. Was the main procedure a laminectomy, laminotomy, or discectomy? _____

   c. How many interspaces were involved? _____

   d. Assign the procedure code(s) for this encounter. _____

8. When assigning codes for pain management injections, the coder should determine the following: **a.** Was the injection for diagnostic or _____ purposes? **b.** Where is the injection being performed, nerve or _____? **c.** _____ is being injected? **d.** For spinal injections, what is the _____ the injection? **e.** Is this a single injection or _____ infusion? **f.** For spinal injection, if it is unilateral or _____. **g.** How many _____?

9. A patient has longstanding numbness, aching pain, and loss of grip in her right hand. Splinting and conservative measures have not resolved her carpal tunnel syndrome. The physician performs carpal tunnel release and, while using the microscope, performs an internal neurolysis. What code(s) will be reported? _____

   _____

10. A patient suffered a laceration of the radial digital nerve of the right ring finger while slicing a bagel. She went to the ED that day; the ED physician suspected nerve damage and referred the patient to the orthopedist. Four days later, upon examination, the orthopedist notes that the patient does have loss of pinpoint touch over the radial aspect of the finger. Surgery is performed the following day by suturing the nerve under microscopic view. Assign the codes for this service. _____

   _____

   _____

CASE STUDIES

1. Trent B.

   Trent was walking on the beach and stepped on a metal shard, severing the superficial branch of the external plantar nerve. He lost sensation along the outer side of the foot. The nerve was repaired by using a nerve graft from the sural nerve. The external digital nerve was restored by suturing the 1.5-cm graft to the proximal and distal ends of the damaged nerve using the operative microscope.

   What code(s) will be reported? _____

   _____

2. Casey Y.

   Casey is experiencing intractable pain to the face and his oral pain medications have not eliminated his pain. The physician feels that destruction of the trigeminal nerve may solve his long-term pain. A neurolytic agent is injected into the trigeminal nerve.

   What code(s) will be reported? _____

   _____

3. Homer T.

   Homer, a 20-year-old male, arrives in the ED with complaints of headache, blurred vision, and left leg pain. He was born with hydrocephalus requiring ventriculoperitoneal shunt of the left lateral ventricle as a newborn. The physician suspects shunt malfunction and orders imaging, which confirms malfunction. The patient undergoes a VP shunt revision with replacement of the shunt.

   Assign the procedure codes for the physician. _____

   _____

4. Mona M.

   Mona has had several series of epidural injections with some success. The neurosurgeon feels that neurostimulator insertion for long-term therapy would be beneficial. Mona is placed in the prone position and a midline incision is made overlying the affected vertebrae. The fascia is divided and the paravertebral muscles are retracted away. The surgeon places the inductive electrode pads in the epidural space proximal to the damaged spinal segment. The pulse generator is sutured over the muscles and the skin is closed.

   Assign the procedure codes for the physician. _____

5. Ho-Sook K.

   > **PREOPERATIVE DIAGNOSIS:** Right ulnar neuropathy.
   > **OPERATIVE PROCEDURE:** Right ulnar nerve neurolysis and transposition.
   > **PROCEDURE DESCRIPTION:** A small curvilinear incision was made in the right elbow, extending above and below the medial epicondyle, and with sharp and blunt dissection the ulnar nerve was exposed. It was found to be scarred down the cubital tunnel and was released gently with sharp and blunt dissection. A vessel loop was used to go around the nerve, and with gentle retraction it was released from the surrounding scar tissue. Intraoperative nerve stimulation was used in order to avoid injuring the motor branches. Enough length of nerve was obtained in order to transpose it across the medial epicondyle on the right. A fascia sling was developed and the nerve was transposed in front of the medial epicondyle. This was to make sure that the nerve was without tension in both flexion and extension. The subcutaneous tissue was closed with #2-0 Vicryl, and the skin was closed with #3-0 running nylon.

   Assign the procedure codes for the physician. _____

   _____

6. Amos T.

PREOPERATIVE DIAGNOSIS: Right lumbosacral radiculopathy secondary to herniations.
PROCEDURE PERFORMED: Right L5 and S1 transforaminal epidural steroid injection.
DESCRIPTION OF PROCEDURE: The right S1 foramen was identified fluoroscopically using AP fluoroscopy. The overlying tissues were then infiltrated with 3 cc of 2% lidocaine. Under fluoroscopic guidance, a 22-gauge, 3.5-inch sterile spinal needle was directed toward the superolateral aspect of the right S1 foramen. Once the needle tip was noted to be in the correct position, and after negative aspiration for CSF or blood, 1 cc of Isovue-200 was instilled followed by 40 mg of Kenalog. The needle was then withdrawn. Attention was then turned to the right L5 foramen overlying tissues, which were identified using a right oblique fluoroscopy. The overlying tissues were infiltrated with 3 cc of 2% lidocaine. Under fluoroscopic guidance, a 22-gauge, 5-inch sterile spinal needle was directed toward the 6 o'clock position of the L5 pedicle. Once the needle tip was noted to be in the correct position and after negative aspiration for CSF or blood, 1 cc of Isovue-200 was instilled, creating a typical L5 radicologram. Then 40 mg of Kenalog were instilled. The needle was then withdrawn. Hemostasis was achieved immediately.

Assign the procedure codes for the physician. _____

_____

7. Radomir R.

OPERATION:
1. Bilateral L2–L3 paravertebral facet block.
2. Bilateral L3–L4 paravertebral facet block.
3. Bilateral L4–L5 paravertebral facet block.
4. Bilateral L5–S1 paravertebral facet block.
5. Fluoroscopic needle localization.
PROCEDURE: Using AP fluoroscopy, the L2 through S1 vertebral levels were easily identified, beginning with the right side of the patient's spine, with a 15-degree oblique positioning to reveal the Scotty dog views. Next, 1% lidocaine was infiltrated into the skin and subcutaneous tissues over the eye of the Scotty dog at L2–L3 on the right, followed by insertion of a 5-inch, 22-gauge sharp Quincke Point needle directed in a gun-barrel fashion under fluoroscopy until contact was made with the upper outer quadrant of the eye of the Scotty dog. After a negative aspiration, 2 cc of 0.25% Bupivacaine and 3 mg of Celestone were injected.
Our attention was then turned to the L3–L4 level on the right where, again, the same procedure was completed. Our attention was then turned to the L4–L5 level, where again, the identical procedure was carried out. Finally, our attention was turned to the L5–S1 level, where the identical procedure was again carried out.
Our attention was then turned to the left side of the patient's spine. The fluoroscope was moved to approximately 15-degree left oblique positioning from midline to reveal the Scotty dog view from L2 to S1 on the left. Beginning at L2–L3, 1% lidocaine was infiltrated into the skin and subcutaneous tissues over the eye of the Scotty dog, followed by the insertion of a 5-inch, 22-gauge sharp Quincke Point needle through the anesthetized skin and directed in a gun-barrel fashion until contact was made with the upper outer quadrant of the eye of the Scotty dog. After a negative aspiration, 2 cc of 0.25% Bupivacaine and 3 mg of Celestone were injected.
Our attention was then turned to the L3–L4 level on the left where, again, 1% lidocaine was infiltrated into the skin and subcutaneous tissues over the eye of the Scotty dog, followed by insertion of a 5-inch, 22-gauge, sharp Quincke Point needle through the anesthetized skin and directed in a gun-barrel fashion until contact was made with the upper outer quadrant of the eye of the Scotty dog at L3–L4 on the left and 2 cc of 0.25% Bupivacaine and 3 mg of Celestone were injected.

Our attention was then turned to the L4–L5 level on the left, where the same procedure was carried out in the exact same detail. Finally, our attention was turned to the L5–S1 level on the left, where the identical procedure is performed. This completed a bilateral 4-level lumbar paravertebral facet block with fluoroscopy guidance and IV sedation.

Assign the procedure codes for the physician. _____

_____

8. Kay V.

OPERATIVE PROCEDURE: Bilateral C5–C6 medial branch block under fluoroscopy.
PROCEDURE DESCRIPTION: The C-arm was put to AP on the neck at C5–C6 levels on both sides. The lateral masses in her neck were identified. Corresponding skin incision sites were marked to reach 5 mm medial to the neck. Then, a 3.5-inch long, 22-gauge spinal needle was inserted under standard fluoroscopy guidance to reach the periosteum 5 mm medial to the neck. After negative aspiration, 0.5 cc of solution was injected at each level. A similar procedure was done on both sides. The skin was then cleaned and Band-Aids were applied.

Assign the procedure codes for the physician. _____

_____

9. Shonna G.

POSTOPERATIVE DIAGNOSIS: Herniated disk left L4–L5 with lumbar radiculopathy.
OPERATIVE PROCEDURE:
1. Lumbar minimally invasive microlaminotomy, medial facetectomy, and foraminotomy, left L4–L5.
2. Minimally invasive left L4–L5 microdiscectomy.
3. Intraoperative fluoroscopy and intraoperative microdissection were used.
PROCEDURE DESCRIPTION: A small incision was made slightly paraspinal to the spinous process to the left. With sharp and blunt dissection, lamina and facets of L4 and L5 were exposed. Intraoperative x-rays were used for localization again, and the minimally invasive retractors were placed in position. The laminotomy was performed with the help of Kerrison punches, and ligamentum flavum was removed. A microscope was brought into the field. After extending the laminotomy and medial facetectomy, decompressing the lateral recess of the part of the ligamentum, the flavum was removed as well. The nerve root was identified and retracted gently without help of cotton paddies. The disk was identified and opened with a #15 blade in a square window shape manner. The discectomy was performed with the help of pituitary rongeurs in various orientations and the disk was irrigated with pressure with a 14-gauge Angiocath and 10-cc syringe.

Assign the procedure codes for the physician. _____

_____

10. Allen E.

Allen is seen for chronic headaches. The physician performs a bilateral suboccipital block. A 22-gauge 1½-inch needle was placed midway between the left occipital protuberance and the left mastoid process. Marcaine and Aristocort were injected in a fanlike fashion to infiltrate the greater and lesser occipital nerves. The same procedure was carried out on the right side.

Assign the procedure codes for the physician. _____

_____

INTERNET RESEARCH

1. Neurostimulators can be inserted for various conditions in addition to pain. Visit the Centers for Medicare and Medicaid Services (CMS) website and search for coverage policies for neurostimulators. For a sacral neurostimulator, what documentation does CMS require for coverage purposes?

2. Visit Human Anatomy Online at www.innerbody.com and click on "Nervous System." Here you can review the components of the nervous system, eyes, and ears. The animations demonstrate the functions of each organ system and also provide tutorials allowing you to participate by clicking on various nerves and body parts, defining what they are and how they work.

3. Visit http://library.med.utah.edu/neurologicexam/cases/home_cases.html and select Menu of Cases. Participate in the interactive Case No. 01, "The Upset Office Manager." You will walk through the history, exam, and medical decision making as would a physician examining this patient. Follow the instructions provided throughout the case. What is the patient's final diagnosis?

MEDICAL CODING LAB Remember to use the coding activities at **Medicalcodinglab.com** for extra practice on what you have just learned and to test your knowledge.

CPT: Eye and Ear

Chapter 26 in *Conquer Medical Coding* explains the correct coding and sequencing of diseases, injuries, and procedures included in the CPT's eye and ear sections. Typical procedures performed on the eye are foreign body removal, cataract removal, glaucoma surgery, laser surgery for vision correction, and plastic and reconstructive surgery of the eye and surrounding structures. Chapter 26 also explains coding for the auditory system, which includes procedures on the external ear, middle ear, inner ear, and temporal bone. The codes are arranged by anatomical part and then by procedure on that part. In addition, Chapter 26 includes the following topics:

- When codes from the eye and ear section of CPT are used versus integumentary for removing lesions of the eyelid
- How to determine when blepharoptosis repair is performed for cosmetic purposes versus a medical condition
- The difference between phototherapeutic keratectomy and photorefractive keratectomy procedures
- The difference between extracapsular and intracapsular cataract extraction and complex cataract extractions
- The difference between tympanostomy and myringotomy for insertion of ventilation tubes
- The purpose and components of tympanoplasty

CODE IT!

Supply the correct codes for the following.

1. _____ A 5-year-old patient with recurrent otitis media has bilateral myringotomy with removal of a ventilation tube on the left and insertion of ventilation tubes bilaterally.

2. _____ The patient complains of trichiasis on the right upper lid. The eyelid was numbed and the area most affected was treated with electrolysis.

3. _____ The patient suffers from tympanic membrane perforation. The ear was exposed and the operating microscope was used for visualization. The perforation was freshened up and a paper patch was placed.

4. _____ The patient bent over to tie his shoes and dislocated his newly implanted intraocular lens. The physician performs a removal and replacement of the intraocular lens, left eye.

5. _____ An adult patient is seen in the ENT office and has a myringotomy with tube insertion under local anesthesia in the left ear.

6. _____ The patient is status post surgery on the left eye and there is still inflammation present. The physician injects a steroid into the subconjunctival space.

7. _____ The patient has been suffering with a weepy right eye for several months. Conservative measures are not successful. Using local anesthetic drops, the physician dilates the lacrimal punctum and lightly irrigates, opening the blocked punctum and allowing drainage.

8. _____ A construction worker, despite wearing safety glasses, got a small metal shard embedded in his left eyelid. The patient is seen for removal of the foreign body with an adjacent tissue transfer.

9. _____ The patient is evaluated in the office for a sense of fullness in the ear and subjective decreased hearing. The physician examined the patient's left ear, which appeared normal. The right ear showed a bug that looked like a cockroach lodged in the ear canal. The bug appeared to be dead. The physician removed the bug and performed copious irrigation.

10. _____ A patient who was not wearing a helmet was in a four-wheeler accident; he was riding through a wooded area and a branch clipped his right ear. The patient had a 2-cm large laceration requiring otoplasty.

MULTIPLE CHOICE

Select the option that best provides the correct code, completes the statement, or answers the question.

1. An established patient is seen in the office for complaints of decreased hearing and cerumen caked on the edge of the left canal. Examination of both ears was performed. It was clear that the patient has impacted cerumen. Physician removes the cerumen by irrigating to loosen the wax, then uses tweezers to remove the large fragments. What is the correct way to code this situation?
   A. 69450–LT
   B. 69200–LT
   C. 69210–LT
   D. 99212

2. Which CPT code would be reported for the repair of an oval window fistula of the right ear?
   A. 69666
   B. 69320
   C. 69666–RT
   D. 69667

3. A physician performs a resection of the temporal bone using an external approach. Which CPT code would be reported?
   A. 69550
   B. 69535
   C. 69970
   D. 69979

4. Which code would be reported for the implantation of a cochlear device with mastoidectomy?
   A. 69715
   B. 69718
   C. 69930
   D. 69949

5. What is the correct code for a radical excision of a right external auditory canal lesion with neck dissection?
   A. 69140
   B. 69145
   C. 69150
   D. 69155

6. The physician performs the insertion of a replacement intraocular lens right eye with ophthalmic endoscope. The patient is status post cataract extraction 5 years ago. What is the correct way to code this situation?
   A. 66986–RT, 69990
   B. 66986–RT, 66990
   C. 66825–RT, 66990
   D. 66985–RT, 66990

7. A patient receives a YAG laser desiccation of a secondary cataract, left eye. What is the correct way to code for this situation?
   A. 66821–LT
   B. 66820
   C. 66820–LT
   D. 66830–LT

8. A patient with right hypotropia is being treated with inferior rectus recession of 2 mm. What is the correct way to code for this situation?
   A. 67311–RT
   B. 67318–RT
   C. 67320–RT
   D. 67314–RT

9. A 59-year-old male with ptosis is admitted for biopsy of the inferior oblique muscle of his left eye to rule out ocular myasthenia. What is the correct way to code for this situation?
   A. 67810–LT
   B. 20206
   C. 20200
   D. 67346–LT

10. A patient with a conjunctival cyst of the left eye is admitted for incision and drainage (I&D). What is the correct way to code for this situation?
    A. 68040–LT
    B. 68020–LT
    C. 68110–LT
    D. 68100–LT

SHORT ANSWER

Answer the following questions.

1. Diagnosis: Otosclerosis, right ear.

   Procedure: Stapedectomy.

   The stapes superstructure was vaporized with the argon laser. A stapedotomy was created in the footplate and a 4.5-mm McGee piston was inserted. A small piece of tissue was harvested from the postauricular crease and placed in the oval window. What is the correct code and modifier for this procedure? _____

   _____

2. A patient has been complaining of fullness in her right ear and decreased hearing. Upon examination, the physician discovered impacted cerumen. The physician uses suction and forceps to remove the impaction. The patient is instructed to use Debrox to prevent impaction in the future. What is the correct code and modifier for this procedure? _____

_____

3. The lacrimal sac of the patient's left eye has an abscess that must be drained in order for the eye to drain properly. The surgeon makes a small incision directly into the lacrimal sac, and the pressure caused by the abscess is relieved as the area drains. The incision is sutured closed. What is the correct code and modifier for this procedure? _____

_____

4. The terms *tympanostomy*, *myringotomy*, and *tympanic ventilation* are commonly confused and relate to the same procedure. Explain what each of these are and how they are similar or different. _____

_____

_____

5. While gardening earlier in the day, the patient was struck in the left eye with the tip of a rose bush branch. The patient immediately rinsed her eye. Now she feels like she has something in her eye and is having pain, so she visits the urgent care center. She is examined there and no foreign material is located, but she is noted to have a small laceration of the sclera. This is treated with tissue glue. What is the correct code and modifier for this procedure? _____

_____

6. Name three elements a coder needs to know before assigning codes for strabismus surgery.

_____

_____

_____

7. Research the following codes and prepare an explanation of the similarities, differences, and when each is used: 66990 and 69990. _____

_____

_____

_____

8. An insulin-dependent patient with retinal microaneurysmal diabetic retinopathy is seen in the ASC for vitrectomy followed by endolaser photocoagulation of the right eye. The vitreous was sucked mechanically from behind the iris. The laser was used to treat retinal disorders in all four retinal quadrants to prevent further retinal hemorrhage. What is the correct code and modifier for this procedure? _____

_____

9. A patient with glaucoma is taken to the procedure room and given retrobulbar local anesthesia. A microscope is positioned and an incision is made in the conjunctiva down to the surgical limbus. A bleb was created by folding down the conjunctiva over the cornea to expose the sclera. A scleral flap was created and raised with a small incision made

into the anterior chamber. A small block of trabecular mesh was removed to create an opening (fistula) to allow aqueous to flow out of the anterior chamber. A peripheral iridectomy was then performed to promote flow of aqueous from the posterior chamber to the anterior chamber. The scleral and conjunctival flaps were then closed. The bleb serves as a reservoir to hold aqueous fluid that flowed out of the anterior chamber through the fistula and beneath the scleral flap to reach the subconjunctival space and then be absorbed naturally. Does this procedure describe a trabeculoplasty or trabeculectomy? Explain your answer. _____

_____

_____

10. Explain how a coder can identify a complex cataract extraction, what information should be recorded in the procedure note, and what code is reported for this service. _____

_____

_____

CASE STUDIES

1. Dorothea G.

   > **DIAGNOSIS:** Advanced uncontrolled primary open angle glaucoma, right eye.
   > **PROCEDURE:** Trabeculectomy with Mitomycin C application. Incision was made 9 mm posterior to the limbus at 11:30 and the sub-Tenon's space was entered. Dissection was carried out. At the 12:00 position, a trabeculectomy flap was constructed. It was shelved anteriorly into the clear cornea. A punch was used to remove trabecular tissue, after which a peripheral iridectomy was performed. The flap was repositioned and sutures were adjusted until an optimal amount of leakage was noted. Mitomycin C 0.5 mg was used on the tip of a Weck sponge for 1 minute and 45 seconds. Healon was introduced into the anterior chamber to pressurize the eye. The conjunctival incision was closed with Vicryl.

   Assign the procedure code(s) for the physician. _____

2. Anton N.

   Anton is seen in the ASC for corneal transplant of the right eye. The cornea is severely scarred from a chemical burn. He had an IOL placed last year. Anesthesia is provided and the eyeball is exposed. The center of the cornea is marked for removal. The donor cornea is then cut to fit. Using a trephine, the cornea is cut. The donor cornea is then placed in the eye and sutured. The eye is patched.

   Assign the procedure code(s) for the physician. _____

3. Norbet U.

   > **DIAGNOSIS:** Nuclear sclerotic cataract extraction of the left eye.
   > **PROCEDURE:** Phacoemulsification with IOL insertion.
   > **DESCRIPTION OF PROCEDURE:** An incision was made in the scleral groove, creating a scleral tunnel. The anterior chamber was entered and a continuous tear capsulotomy was performed. The nucleus was hydrodissected and phacoemulsification was carried out in the posterior chamber. Healon was inserted into the anterior chamber. A foldable IOL was placed in the posterior chamber and sealed.

   Assign the procedure code(s) for the physician. _____

4. Amanda P.

> **PROCEDURE:** Chalazion of the right upper lid.
> **DESCRIPTION OF PROCEDURE:** A clamp placed on the lid was inverted. The tarsal surface was incised to gain access to the sac. I&D of the chalazion was performed, after which the sac and its material were resected. The same technique was performed on the other chalazion. TobraDex ointment was applied.

Assign the procedure code(s) for the physician. _____

5. Keesha A.

Pterygium of the right eye is excised with conjunctival autograft with superficial keratotomy. She has a peripheral progressive pterygium that has moved into the visual axis. The eye is prepped and the operating microscope is used in excising the pterygium. The scar tissue is scraped away from the cornea and limbus. A burr is used to smooth the corneal surface and limbus and a Tenon's fascia is removed away to within 2 mm of the corneal limbus. A 5 × 7 × 7 free conjunctival graft is harvested from the superior conjunctiva.

Assign the procedure code(s) for the physician. _____

6. Daniel O.

Daniel has chronic otitis media with a longstanding history of drainage from the TM. A posterior canal skin flap is made. A canaloplasty is performed to allow exposure. A small atticotomy is made to expose the ossicular chain. The incus is completely eroded. The malleous is left to be used to anchor the reconstruction. The stapes is frozen from tympanosclerosis. The stapes is mobilized, picking away at the calcific tympanosclerosis. Tympanoplasty is performed and Gelfoam and the fascia graft are placed under the malleous remnant. The fascia graft is obtained and placed under the malleus remnant.

Assign the procedure code(s) for the physician. _____

7. Chandler L.

Chandler, an 11-year-old autistic child, is seen for otological examination under anesthesia. He suffers from chronic ear infection and is uncooperative for examination in the office. His right ear is examined and the canal is cleaned of debris. A myringotomy is performed with placement of a PE tube. The left ear is also examined and the canal cleaned of debris. The TM appears pink and without effusion.

Assign the procedure code(s) for the physician. _____

8. Thomas E.

> **DIAGNOSIS:** Type II tympanic membrane perforation and conductive hearing loss, right ear.
> **PROCEDURE:** Ossicular exploration and cartilage inlay graft.
> Cerumen was removed from the external auditory canal. A microscope was used to visualize the inner ear. The perforation was identified and the edges were freshened using a pick and stapes curette. The ossicles were examined and palpated. All components of the inner ear moved well. A cartilage graft from the tragus was obtained and cut into a round shape to cover the 4 × 5 mm perforation in the tympanum. Drops and a cotton ball were placed and the procedure was ended.

Assign the procedure code(s) for the physician. _____

9. Bai C.

Bai presented with esotropia and was admitted to the ASC for recession of the medial rectus muscle, bilaterally. He was taken to the OR and prepped and draped. An incision was made through the conjunctiva and Tenon's capsule of the right eye. The medial rectus muscle was then isolated using three muscle hooks. The pole test was performed to ensure the entire muscle was hooked. A double-armed 8-0 Vicyrl suture was then used to suture the muscle with locking bites at each end. The muscle was then detached from the globe and the suture was inspected and found to be intact. Hemostasis was achieved using bipolar cautery. The muscle was reattached to the sclera 4.0 mm posterior to the original insertion site. Attention was turned to the left medial rectus muscle recession and the same procedure was carried out on that side.

Assign the procedure code(s) for the physician. _____

10. Billy C.

> **PROCEDURE:** Entropion repair with base down triangular wedge tarsal resection, right lower lid.
> **DESCRIPTION OF PROCEDURE:** Billy received a local injection of Marcaine, Xylocaine with Wydase under IV pentothal sedation, through local infiltration of the right lower lid. He was then prepped and draped in the usual manner. A large chalazion clamp in the temporal right lower lid area was then everted and a base down triangle was made approximately 6 x 6 x 6 mm with the apex near the lash margin. This was removed with a Bard-Parker and sharp dissection, causing a resection of the tarsal plate and subconjunctival tissue. Three separate 6-0 black silk sutures were used to bring the edges together, causing a pocketing of the right lower lid. Maxitrol ointment was applied. Eye dressing with an eye pad was placed.

Assign the procedure code(s) for the physician. _____

INTERNET RESEARCH

1. Visit Otolaryngology Houston's website at www.ghorayeb.com/Pictures.html to view pictures of ear anatomy and tympanoplasty and mastoidectomy procedures.
2. Visit the Ophthalmology Unit, Universiti Malaysia Sarawak, website at www.sarawakeyecare.com. Select "Case of the Week" and choose three cases to code.
3. Visit these specialty society websites and look for coding-related material on any of the topics discussed in this chapter: American Academy of Otolaryngology–Head and Neck Surgery (http://entnet.org) and American Academy of Ophthalmology (www.aao.org). (*Hint:* Use the quick link for "Young Ophthalmologists" as one area to locate coding instruction.)

MEDICAL CODING LAB Remember to use the coding activities at **Medicalcodinglab.com** for extra practice on what you have just learned and to test your knowledge.

CPT: Radiology Codes

Chapter 27 in *Conquer Medical Coding* explains the basic CPT radiology and other imaging coding. The radiology section has seven subsections organized according to method or type of radiology and its purpose, including diagnostic and interventional radiology mammography, nuclear medicine, and ultrasound. Understanding the difference between modalities such as radiological examination (x-ray), CT scan, MRI scan, and MRA scan is essential to determining the correct code for radiology services. Codes are assigned using the physician orders, test requisitions, and ancillary reports documentation. Chapter 27 also explains the following topics:

- The key guidelines for the radiology section
- The code selection for radiology procedures that use or do not use contrast material
- The difference between the professional and technical components of radiology services and how to designate this by using modifiers
- The correct assignment of radiological supervision and interpretation services
- The difference between diagnostic imaging and interventional radiology procedures

CODE IT!

Assign all pertinent procedure codes, modifiers, and HCPCS codes.

1. _____ X-ray, left elbow with four views, complete

2. _____ Diagnostic nuclear medicine procedure for thyroid imaging with vascular flow

3. _____ Abdominal ultrasound, real time, limited

4. _____ Unlisted CPT code for therapeutic radiology clinical treatment planning

5. _____ Ultrasound of the chest, real time with image documentation

6. _____ Therapeutic radiology simulation-aided field setting; complex

7. _____ Chest x-ray with two views of lateral and frontal with fluoroscopy

8. _____ Bilateral screening mammography in a 48-year-old

9. _____ CT scan of the head with contrast material by radiology clinic (include modifier)

10. _____ AP view of the pelvis and AP and oblique views of the hips

MULTIPLE CHOICE

Select the option that best provides the correct code, completes the statement, or answers the question.

1. A patient receives an ultrasound at 23 weeks' gestation transabdominally to determine placental location. What is the correct way to code this situation?
   A. 76815
   B. 76805
   C. 76817
   D. 76811

2. Injection of contrast for a left ankle arthrography is reported by the physician who performed both the procedure and the interpretation. What is the correct way to code this situation?
   A. 73615
   B. 73615, 27648
   C. 27648–LT, 73615–LT–51
   D. 73600

3. A patient receives a myelography S&I, cervical, complete with injection procedure. What is the correct way to code this situation?
   A. 62284
   B. 62302
   C. 72240
   D. 62284, 62302

4. A patient diagnosed with breast cancer undergoes mastectomy and chemotherapy. She receives radiation treatment delivery to the right breast area at 4 MeV. What is the correct way to code this situation?
   A. 77407
   B. 77401
   C. 77412
   D. 77402

5. An asymptomatic patient is seen for her routine annual screening mammogram. Radiology report shows microcalcifications on the left. What is the correct way to code this situation?
   A. 77053–50
   B. 77066
   C. 77059
   D. 77067

6. A patient eating at a restaurant began feeling like something was stuck in her throat. She is seen in the ED and the physician orders an x-ray of her throat. The diagnosis is embedded distal esophageal foreign body. What is the correct way to code this situation?
   A. 74240
   B. 74210
   C. 74220
   D. 70360

7. If a screening mammogram is performed followed by a diagnostic mammogram on the same day, which modifier is reported?
   A. –59
   B. –51
   C. –GG
   D. –GH

8. Select the correct code for cardiac MRI, without contrast, with stress imaging.
   A. 75563
   B. 75561
   C. 75557
   D. 75559

9. A 6-year-old patient with a history of urinary incontinence and UTI is seen for a nuclear ureteral reflux study followed by bladder residual study. What is the correct way to code this situation?
   A. 78761, 78730
   B. 78740, 78730
   C. 78740
   D. 78725, 78730

10. Per CPT guidelines, which of the following is the definition of "report" as it relates to results, tests, and interpretations?
   A. Reports are the work product of the interpretation of numerous test results.
   B. Reports lead to results.
   C. Reports are the technical component of a service.
   D. Reports lead to interpretation.

SHORT ANSWER

Answer the following questions.

1. Name the two modes and two scan definitions of diagnostic ultrasound.

   a. _____

   _____

   b. _____

   _____

2. A 50-year-old post-hysterectomy female taking Prednisone undergoes a dual energy x-ray absorptiometry body composition exam. The patient lies on the examination table, and the central DXA unit measures bone density of the hips, pelvis, and lower spine. Assign the code(s).

   _____

3. Research the CMS coverage policy for bone mineral density for screening and monitoring DEXA (or DXA) scans and answer the following questions:

   a. What CPT codes are reported for screening DEXA? _____

   _____

   _____

   b. What CPT codes are reported for DEXA for monitoring? _____

   _____

c. Are there specific coverage criteria for when these are recommended and medically appropriate? List your source and what the criteria are for screening DEXA and DEXA for monitoring purposes. _____

_____

_____

_____

4. Search the Internet for *ACR Practice Parameter for Communication of Diagnostic Imaging Findings* and answer the following questions:

a. Is it appropriate for a nonphysician to provide an interpretation or final impression of the film or study performed? _____

b. List the main components of the report as recommended by ACR. _____

_____

_____

_____

_____

_____

5. Can coders assign diagnosis or procedure codes from a radiology report? Research trusted sources such as CMS, AHIMA, and AAPC and explain your answer. _____

_____

_____

6. A radiology report must be accessible and present in the record before a coder may assign the procedure code and subsequent modifier –26. Name the elements that the CPT manual says are required of the report. _____

_____

_____

7. How does a coder determine if a radiologist should report a screening mammography or a diagnostic mammography code? _____

_____

_____

8. Explain why identifying the views obtained or the patient's position when imaging is performed is relevant to procedure code assignment. _____

_____

_____

9. What is the code for an x-ray of the mandible on both sides of the face? Would modifier –50 be reported? Why or why not? _____

_____

10. What source is used to confirm if a procedure code has a professional and technical component allotted or if a procedure is considered bilateral or not? Where is this located? _____

_____

_____

CASE STUDIES

1. Chas M.

   Chas is diagnosed with an inoperable endobronchial tumor. Following localization radiographs, HDR brachytherapy treatment is administered. A remote afterloader guides the iridium-192 source into position, 1 channel.

   Assign the code for the facility. _____

2. Alma A.

   > **INDICATION:** Abdominal pain and constipation.
   > **X-RAY:** Flat plate of abdomen. The patient complains of left lower abdominal pain and constipation.
   > **INTERPRETATION:** The intestinal gas pattern is normal. There is no evidence for obstruction or ileus. No masses or abnormal calcifications are identified at this time.
   > **ASSESSMENT:** Normal flat plate of abdomen.

   a. *Assign the procedure code for the radiologist.* _____

   b. *Assign the procedure code for the facility.* _____

3. Cleavon G.

   The physician orders a computed tomography (CT) of the pelvis for a patient with recurrent diverticulitis and abdominal pain to confirm a suspected diagnosis of Crohn's disease.

   > **PROCEDURE:** Oral contrast is given and 120 cc of Omnipaque is power injected via IV. Images are obtained from the iliac crest to the symphysis pubis.
   > There is marked diverticulosis of the sigmoid colon and rectum. All signs of activity are seen in the form of ileal wall thickening, intense wall enhancement, mesenteric fat stranding, and comb sign of the mesenteric vessels denoting mesenteric engorgement.
   > **IMPRESSION:** Diverticulosis; Crohn's disease.

   a. *Assign the procedure code for the radiologist.* _____

   b. *Assign the procedure code for the facility.* _____

4. Ty K.

   Ty, a corrections officer with left shoulder pain and instability, is seen in outpatient testing for arthrography, arthrogram, and MRI with contrast. (Cases 4 to 6 are for the same patient.)

   > Scout view radiograph images of the shoulder were obtained last week. Using fluoroscopic guidance, the glenohumeral joint was punctured with a 22-gauge spinal needle. Contrast is injected to successfully confirm placement of the needle position. Next, approximately 20 cc of saline, gadolinium, and iodinated contrast was injected into the joint space. The patient tolerated the procedure well.
   > **IMPRESSION:** Joint injection for radiographic arthrography and MR arthrogram.

   a. *Assign the procedure code for the radiologist.* _____

   b. *Assign the procedure code for the facility.* _____

5. Ty K.

> The patient received a left shoulder arthrogram.
> Joint images were obtained a week ago. Additional radiographs were obtained after the injection. These scout view images showed an osseous abnormality. There was no extravasation of contrast into the subacromial or subdeltoid bursa indicating rotator cuff tear. No abnormalities were identified.
> **IMPRESSION:** Negative shoulder arthrogram.

a. *Assign the procedure code for the radiologist.* _____

b. *Assign the procedure code for the facility.* _____

6. Ty K.

> Following the arthrogram, the patient was taken to the MRI suite for imaging with contrast with T1, T2, and fat-suppressed sequences in axial, oblique, coronal, and sagittal projections. The supraspinatus and other rotator cuff tendons appear normal, including the glenoid labrum and capsule. No osseous lesions were noted.
> **IMPRESSION:** Negative MRI examination of left shoulder.

a. *Assign the procedure code for the radiologist.* _____

b. *Assign the procedure code for the facility.* _____

7. Tilda S.

Tilda, a 52-year-old patient with renal cancer with acute lateral and lumbar spine pain, is seen in outpatient testing for skeletal scintigram.

> **PROCEDURE:** Total body scanning was carried out in anterior and posterior views, 2 hours following the administration of Tc 99, mdp.
> Examination reveals a significant trace of accumulation in the L5 vertebral body and also in the right 8th rib laterally. There are no other skeletal lesions identified. Renal and bladder images are present as expected.
> **IMPRESSION:** Focal abnormalities at the body of L5 and the 8th rib laterally. Changes are compatible with recent healing fractures. The pattern does not suggest metastatic disease.

a. *Assign the procedure code for the radiologist.* _____

b. *Assign the procedure code for the facility.* _____

8. Cassie K.

Cassie is seen in the urologist office for renal ultrasound.

> **INTERPRETATION:** Both kidneys are well seen and normal in size. The right kidney measures 11.8 cm in length and the left 12.4 cm in length. No hydronephrosis or focal masses are seen. Cortical thickness and echogenicity are normal.
> **IMPRESSION:** Normal renal ultrasound.

Assign the procedure code for the urologist. _____

9. Michael D.

Michael, a male patient with prostate cancer, is seen in the outpatient nuclear medicine department for placement of radioactive seeds for prostate brachytherapy. Simulation was performed to determine the field setting and placement of seeds; 70 seeds of iodine-125 were inserted using ultrasound guidance.

a. *Assign the radiology codes only.* _____

b. *Assign the procedure code for the radiologist.* _____

c. *Assign the procedure code for the facility.* _____

10. Mai L.

Mai tripped at home climbing up the steps and injured her nose and right shoulder. She went to her local urgent care center for evaluation.

> **PROCEDURE:** X-ray of nasal bones.
> There is an acute and minimally displaced fracture of the nasal bones. There is no gross deviation of the nasal septum. Paranasal sinuses appear normal.
> **IMPRESSION:** Acute and minimally displaced fracture of the nasal bones.
> **PROCEDURE:** Shoulder minimum two views, right shoulder.
> **IMPRESSION:** AP, axillary, and outlet projections of the shoulder demonstrate the boney structures to be intact. The shoulder space is maintained as well as the subacromial space.

a. *Assign the procedure codes for the radiologist.* _____

b. *Assign the procedure codes for the facility.* _____

INTERNET RESEARCH

1. Visit the website of the American Society for Therapeutic Radiology and Oncology at https://www.astro.org/Coding. Navigate through "Coding Guidance" and "Coding FAQs and Tips/ to learn more about brachytherapy. Read the information, and explain the difference between low-dose and high-dose therapy. What coding tips are provided for coding interstitial brachytherapy? What items does the site note that Medicare does not pay for?

2. Visit the American Community of Cancer Centers' website at https://www.accc-cancer.org/ossn_network/and search for "Oncology Reimbursement Update." Read the latest PDF.

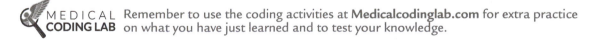 Remember to use the coding activities at **Medicalcodinglab.com** for extra practice on what you have just learned and to test your knowledge.

CHAPTER 28

CPT: Pathology and Laboratory Codes

Chapter 28 in *Conquer Medical Coding* explains the difference between the professional and technical components of the pathology and laboratory medicine services. The technical component encompasses the allocation of staff and technologists, use of equipment, processing and developing of film, injection of the contrast material, and related pre- and post-injection services. The professional component encompasses the physician's time and skill in reading and interpreting the test and providing a written report rendering his or her opinion, advice, or assessment of findings. The physician orders test requisitions and reviews laboratory reports to build a complete clinical picture of a patient's workup and assign procedure codes. With the exception of pathology reports, these documents are never used to assign diagnosis codes. In addition, Chapter 28 covers the following topics:

- When a pathology or laboratory service requires the modifier –26 or modifier –TC
- The specific coding rules associated with reporting panel codes
- The distinction between qualitative and quantitative drug testing
- The basis for code selection in molecular pathology
- When one or more pathology codes are needed based on the specimens received by the surgical pathology department
- The different types of pathology consultation services

CODE IT!

1. _____ Blood gas measurement, pH, and CO_2

2. _____ Clinical diagnosis: Torn meniscus. Tissue submitted: Meniscus, left knee. Gross and microscopic examination performed

3. _____ Obstetric panel

4. _____ Urinalysis, microscopic only

5. _____ Testosterone, total

6. _____ Creatinine, blood

7. _____ Semen analysis, complete

8. _____ Peripheral blood smear interpretation by physician with a written report

9. _____ Amniocentesis for alpha-fetoprotein analysis

10. _____ Pathologist examined the following specimen: Examination was both gross and microscopic; prostate, radical resection

MULTIPLE CHOICE

Select the option that best provides the correct code, completes the statement, or answers the question.

1. A mother brings her son to the pediatrician's office with a sore throat. A strep A infection is suspected. The physician performs an analysis using a rapid identification diagnosis kit. What is the correct way to code this situation?
   A. 87650
   B. 87880
   C. 87652
   D. 87653

2. A blood sample was obtained at the internist office for a lipid panel for a non-Medicare patient. The specimen was sent to an outside laboratory for testing, analysis, and interpretation. The office has a purchased technical contract arrangement with Labquest. What is the correct way to code this situation?
   A. 36415
   B. 80061
   C. 80061–90
   D. 36415, 80061–90

3. The physician orders a urinalysis for a patient with hematuria. The laboratory performs a concentration method and prepares slides for the pathologist to read. The pathologist's findings reveal abnormal cells indicative of transitional cell carcinoma of the bladder. What is the correct way to code this situation?
   A. 88108
   B. 88104
   C. 87015
   D. 87088

4. What is the correct way to code for prothrombin time and activated partial thromboplastin time?
   A. 85610, 85730
   B. 85670, 85730
   C. 85611, 85670
   D. 85730, 85670

5. What is the correct way to code for paternity testing?
   A. 86900
   B. 86910
   C. 86920
   D. 86904

6. What codes are reported when a provider orders the following tests: CBC automated with manual differential, TSH, comprehensive metabolic panel, uric acid, sed rate (automated), fluorescent ANA, and Rh factor?
   A. 80053, 80050, 85652, 86038
   B. 86431, 86255, 80050, 84520
   C. 80050, 86431, 85652, 86038, 84550
   D. 85651, 86255, 80050, 86038

7. What is the correct way to code for gross and microscopic examination of the kidney specimen from a total resection procedure?
   A. 88306
   B. 88307
   C. 88300
   D. 88305

8. What is the correct way to code for surgical pathology examination of bone marrow biopsy?
   A. 88307
   B. 88309
   C. 88172
   D. 88305

9. What is the correct way to code for identification of the amount of digoxin in the blood (quantitative)?
   A. 80375
   B. 80305
   C. 80162
   D. 80299

10. The patient was treated as an outpatient for cellulitis of the leg. He did not respond to treatment and required inpatient hospitalization for intravenous antibiotics. The culture was positive for methicillin-resistant *staphylococcus aureus* (MRSA). What is the correct way to code this situation?
    A. 87641
    B. 87880
    C. 87903
    D. 87640

SHORT ANSWER

1. When a laboratory drug test is qualitative, it measures the _____ of the drug.

2. How many levels of surgical pathology are there? _____

3. In pathology, the number of specimens received in the lab is only one aspect of assigning the number of units for billing. What else must be considered to accurately reflect the number of units that may be billed? _____

   _____

   _____

4. What is FOBT? What code is assigned for FOBT, two determinations? What are Medicare guidelines for ordering, performing, and reporting this test? _____

   _____

   _____

5. A patient is seen for a screening Pap smear. Cervical Pap is screened automatically by the machine and then manually evaluated by the physician with interpretation. The results were abnormal. What code does the laboratory report? After receiving a report of an abnormal Pap smear 2 weeks ago, the patient presents in the office today for diagnostic colposcopy with biopsy of the cervix to rule out cervical dysplasia. What pathology code is reported? _____

   _____

   _____

6. A chemotherapy patient suffering from anemia secondary to treatment presents to his oncologist's office for his routine vitamin B_{12} injection for vitamin B_{12} deficiency anemia due to chemotherapy. While he is there, he also has his CBC drawn, which is sent to an outside lab for processing, and has a finger stick to check his hemoglobin. What codes will the office report? What codes will the lab report? _____

_____

_____

7. A patient is scheduled for a laparoscopically assisted vaginal hysterectomy (LAVH), and the hospital pathologist has been asked to stand by for immediate frozen section availability if there is any concern as to whether or not the leiomyoma are cancerous. The surgery takes 2 hours; the pathologist is on standby for 40 minutes. The pathologist receives the uterus and performs gross and microscopic analysis. The final pathology report and the attending physician confirm the diagnosis of endometriosis of the uterus. What codes will the pathologist report? _____

_____

8. Medicare requires HCPCS codes when available for procedures and services and these supersede existing CPT codes. What codes are reported when performing drug screenings on Medicare patients? _____

_____

9. When performing ancillary testing, it is a requirement that the lab or pathologist obtain what before proceeding with testing? _____

_____

_____

10. CMS has strict rules for assigning diagnosis codes for ancillary tests ordered. The requirements vary depending on which fee schedule the code for the test resides on and is reimbursed from the Medicare Physician Fee Schedule (MPFS) or Clinical Laboratory Fee Schedule (CLFS). What is the key difference that drives how a coder assigns the diagnosis codes? Reference the following sources to locate your answers: Balanced Budget Act of 1997 Section 4317, IOM Chapter 15, Section 80, and Clinical Laboratory Improvement Act of 1988 to find your answer. _____

_____

_____

CASE STUDIES

1. Andrew C.

   Andrew, a 19-year-old male, is involved in a single car motor vehicle accident (MVA). The situation is unclear, but it appears that the patient is under the influence of alcohol or drugs. Police discover a bag of brightly colored pills thought to be "Ecstasy." The ED physician orders an alcohol screening; because of the pills, he also orders a drug screen (multiclass one phase). The presence of methamphetamine and alcohol is noted, and drug confirmation is performed.

   Assign the lab codes for this case. _____

212   Part III: CPT and HCPCS Coding   *CPT* © 2017 American Medical Association, All Rights Reserved.

2. Carmine O.

Carmine, a cystic fibrosis patient, has been fighting a respiratory infection and was prescribed Tobramycin. She must have her Tobramycin level checked monthly.

Assign the laboratory codes for this case. _____

3. Janessa N.

Janessa presented with a cough, fever, and dyspnea. Chest x-ray was positive for a left lower lobe infiltrate. Sputum fluorescent smear and culture was positive for *Haemophilus influenzae* (*H influenzae*).

Assign the codes for the sputum culture and smear. _____

4. Wanda J.

Wanda is admitted for a total knee replacement for her osteoarthritis. After surgery, she develops anemia and sepsis. In anticipation of a transfusion, the lab performs blood antigen screening for compatibility. She is treated with leukocyte transfusion.

What codes will the facility report? _____

5. Norma A.

After observing that a spot on her upper leg had grown bigger, a patient sees her dermatologist. The dermatologist suspects malignancy and excises the 3.3-cm spot, followed by a simple closure. The pathologist performs gross and microscopic review and determines it is basal cell carcinoma.

Assign the pathology code. _____

6. Don H.

> **PATHOLOGY REPORT**
> **SPECIMEN:** Colon-descending polyp.
> **GROSS DESCRIPTION:** Specimen container labeled "colon descending" consisting of single fragment of light tan mucosal tissue measuring 0.3 cm in greatest dimension.
> **MICROSCOPIC DESCRIPTION:** Sections from the large bowel revealed tubular adenoma. It is characterized by having crypts that have crowded, mildly pseudostratified nuclei with a decrease in the number of goblet cells, and increased numbers of mitoses.

Assign the pathology code. _____

7. Herbert Y.

> **PATHOLOGY REPORT**
> **SPECIMENS:**
> A. Lateral margin left hemimandibular cyst
> B. Anterior mucosal margin
> C. Posterior margin
> **GROSS DESCRIPTION:**
> A. Received in formalin marked Cassette A is a single 1.3 × 0.5 × 0.2 cm irregular pale-grey-tan-to-brown smooth and somewhat fragmented portion of tissue.

B. Received in formalin marked Cassette B is an anterior mucosal margin of 0.8 × 0.2 × 0.15 cm irregular pale-tan fragmented portion of tissue. The frozen section residue is wrapped in biopsy paper.

C. Received fresh frozen section marked Cassette C is a posterior margin of 0.4 × 0.4 × 0.1 cm irregular pale-grey smooth to slightly wrinkled tissue.

MICROSCOPIC DIAGNOSIS:

A. Left lateral margin: Squamous mucosa with a small area of microinvasive squamous cell carcinoma.

B. Anterior mucosal margin: Inflamed squamous mucosa, negative for malignancy.

C. Posterior margin: Inflamed squamous mucosa, negative for malignancy.

FROZEN SECTION DIAGNOSIS:

A. Benign-appearing squamous mucosa. No malignancy seen.

B. Benign-appearing squamous mucosa. No malignancy seen.

COMMENT: Specimens B and C received for intraoperative consultation diagnosis show inflamed squamous mucosa with no evidence of carcinoma. Specimen A shows microscopic nests of well-differentiated squamous cell carcinoma involving the upper lamina propria.

a. *How many specimens are there?* _____

b. *For the frozen sections, how many first tissue blocks were obtained?* _____

c. *Was an intraoperative consultation performed?* _____

d. *Assign the pathology codes.* _____

8. Clyde N.

PATHOLOGY REPORT

SPECIMEN: Atrophic left testicle.

GROSS DESCRIPTION: Formalin container labeled "undescended left testicle" is a single 2.1 × 0.6 × 0.3 cm irregular tan-pink to light purple, slightly roughened, soft, rubbery portion of tissue. The specimen is serially sectioned, wrapped in biopsy paper, and submitted in a single cassette.

DIAGNOSIS:

1. Segment of vas deferens showing marked calcification in adjacent fibrous connective tissue stroma.

2. Small focus of epithelium suggestive of residual rete testis.

Assign the pathology code. _____

9. Josephine E.

PATHOLOGY REPORT

SPECIMEN: Thyroid cyst.

GROSS DESCRIPTION: Received in formalin in a container of 2.7 × 1.6 × 1.5 cm elongated, thin-walled cyst which has a small amount of attached fat. The cyst is intact. It contains red-brown fluid. The wall is smooth. One cassette.

MICROSCOPIC DIAGNOSIS:

1. Cystic papillary carcinoma of the thyroid.

2. Multiple lymphoid aggregates intermingled with neoplastic epithelium.

Assign the pathology code. _____

10. Bhumika R.

> **PATHOLOGY REPORT**
> **CLINICAL DATA:** Fresh specimen R/O tumor.
> **OPERATING ROOM GROSS CONSULTATION:** Breast mass consistent with fibroadenoma.
> **BREAST MASS:** Consistent with fibroadenoma.
> **SPECIMEN:** Right breast mass.
> **GROSS DESCRIPTION:** Received fresh for gross evaluation 2.0 gm 2.0 × 1.7 × 1.2 cm tan-to-pink-tan portion of tissue. The surgical margins are marked with black ink. The specimen is sectioned showing a well-defined 1.6 × 1.5 × 1.0 cm nodule.

Assign the pathology code. _____

INTERNET RESEARCH

1. Visit Medicare's Claims Processing Manual, Chapter 16 at www.cms.gov/Regulations-and-Guidance/Guidance/Manuals/downloads/clm104c16.pdf. How many NCDs does it say there are for clinical diagnostic laboratory services?
2. Visit Medica's site and read their policy: https://www.medica.com/ and search for "laboratory services policy modifier 90." Will Medica reimburse claims with the −90 modifier appended? Explain why or why not.

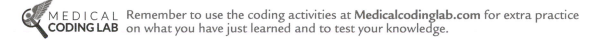 Remember to use the coding activities at **Medicalcodinglab.com** for extra practice on what you have just learned and to test your knowledge.

CHAPTER 29

CPT: Medicine Codes

The Medicine section of CPT is unique in that it includes codes for services that are primarily evaluative and diagnostic in nature. However, it also includes codes for noninvasive or minimally invasive (primarily percutaneous access) services that are not considered surgical, pathology, laboratory, or radiology services. Many of the medicine CPT codes, with the exception of cardiovascular and ophthalmology codes, are associated with primary care practices that provide services and treatments to patients with a variety of medical problems. Chapter 29 in *Conquer Medical Coding* explains the steps for assigning codes for these procedures, including the following topics:

- The conventions specific to administering immunizations and immune globulins
- The difference between infusion and injection, and the rules for properly reporting these services
- ESRD codes based on time factor and physician assessments
- Cardiography tests and their purposes
- The coding conventions for coding the components of cardiac catheterization procedures, including appending HCPCS Level II modifiers as appropriate
- Coding for allergy and clinical immunology services
- The difference between the electrodiagnostic studies of EEG and EMG
- The chemotherapy administration codes and circumstances in which additional codes are appropriate to reflect services provided
- When moderate sedation can be reported separately from the surgical procedure performed
- The rules for coding and reporting assessment and management services on the telephone and Internet by nonphysician staff members

CODE IT!

Assign all pertinent procedure codes, modifiers, and HCPCS codes for the following.

1. _____ An 18-month-old patient is seen by the nurse in the office for his monthly intramuscular injection of RSV immune globulin.

2. _____ A 59-year-old female presents to her family practitioner's office for the intramuscular injection of her annual trivalent, split virus flu vaccine.

3. _____ A call comes in at 8 p.m. from an established patient who needs an E/M service immediately. What medicine code can you report with the E/M code to indicate that services were provided after normal office hours?

4. _____ A frantic mother brings her toddler to her pediatrician after the child ingests liquid Tilex. The pediatrician gives the child ipecac to induce vomiting. Do not assign the E/M code.

5. _____ A 23-year-old patient is exposed to the shingles virus. She has never been vaccinated against varicella zoster. She receives one dose of varicella immune globulin intramuscularly (IM).

6. _____ A patient receives intralesional chemotherapy administration; eight lesions are injected.

7. _____ A physician provides ESRD services for a 55-year-old male over a full month in an outpatient setting with three face-to-face physician visits during the month.

8. _____ A patient is seen 10 days after major surgery for a follow-up visit included in the global service period. How is the visit reported?

9. _____ A patient with ventricular arrhythmia undergoes a microvolt T-wave Alternans test in the outpatient cardiology department.

10. _____ The patient is diagnosed with coronary thrombus; IV infusion of Eminase is performed for thrombolysis of the clot.

MULTIPLE CHOICE

Select the option that best provides the correct code, completes the statement, or answers the question.

1. A patient goes to her doctor's office and receives an injection of 100 mg amikacin sulfate IM for treatment of bacterial colitis. Which of the following codes are reported?
   A. 96372, J0278
   B. 99211, S0072
   C. 96372, J0278 × 2
   D. 99211, J0278 × 2

2. Right heart catheterization is performed in the hospital catheterization lab with coronary angiography and percutaneous coronary thrombolysis via IV infusion. Which of the following codes are reported?
   A. 93456, 92977–51
   B. 93456–26, 92977–51
   C. 93453, 93454
   D. 93453–26, 93454–26

3. A patient presents to her physician to discuss her vaccination history. She is working in the central sterile department of the hospital and is concerned about blood exposure. Her doctor recommends that she receive the hepatitis A and B vaccine intramuscularly. How is this service reported?
   A. 90471, 99211, 90645
   B. 90471, 90636
   C. 90636
   D. 90471, 99212, 90636

4. A patient has MS and is experiencing severe vertigo. She is extremely nauseous and has been vomiting for 2 days. She is now dehydrated and requires electrolytes. The physician orders lactated Ringer's and injection of Phenergan. Infusion time is 65 minutes. Phenergan 50 mg is injected through the IV hep-lock. Which of the following codes are reported?
   A. 96360, +96361, J2550
   B. 96360, 96374, J2550
   C. 96360 × 2, J2550
   D. 96360, 96365, Q0169

5. A patient is seen today for follow up of mitral valve disease. She has valve prolapse and is taking medication. The patient is beginning to have swelling in the lower extremities. Evaluation performed includes 2-D color flow imaging, Doppler exam, and ejection fraction. Overall, the left ventricle is slightly dilated with no wall abnormality. Overall systolic function is borderline normal with ejection fraction at 48%. The right ventricle is normal with normal function. There is moderate right atrial enlargement and gross left atrial enlargement. The aortic valve is normal, whereas the mitral valve is diseased with significant 5+ regurgitation. What type of procedure is this report describing?
   A. Electrocardiogram
   B. Ventriculogram
   C. Electroencephalogram
   D. Echocardiogram

6. A patient is in severe respiratory distress and goes to his physician's office to be seen emergently. The physician's schedule is full except for the emergency slot kept open for any emergency cases that come in. How will the physician report this service?
   A. E/M code
   B. E/M code and 99058
   C. 99060
   D. E/M code with modifier –22

7. A 72-year-old female was admitted to the hospital after suffering diaphoresis, shortness of breath, and heart palpitations while mopping her floor. ECHO showed left ventricular dysfunction with moderate atrial regurgitation; Pacerone therapy and cardioversion were recommended. Direct current external atrial cardioversion was carried out. Which of the following codes is reported?
   A. 93741
   B. 92961
   C. 33211
   D. 92960

8. A 49-year-old ESRD patient is in the hospital August 27 to 30 with stomach flu. She is dehydrated and at high risk because of chronic renal failure. She had been treated for dialysis up until August 26 for her ESRD and dialysis. How is the ESRD service reported for the month of August?
   A. 90957
   B. 90960
   C. 90970 × 26
   D. 90967 × 28

9. A patient with large B-cell cancer is seen in the cancer center for chemotherapy. Neurovista is injected into the subarachnoid space at L1–L2, requiring spinal puncture. Which of the following codes is reported?
   A. 96450
   B. 96542
   C. 96420
   D. 96401

10. A 59-year-old patient was seen in the urologist's office for percutaneous drainage of a renal abscess (50021). The patient could not tolerate the procedure with local anesthesia. The physician administered sedation, and an independently trained nurse observer monitored the patient's level of consciousness for 15 minutes. How is the moderate sedation reported?
   A. 99151
   B. 99152
   C. Do not report moderate sedation
   D. 99153

SHORT ANSWER

Answer the following questions.

1. Under what circumstances can a physician bill for an office E/M visit in addition to allergen immunotherapy codes? _____

2. Which CPT modifier is used with code 92235 performed on both eyes? _____
   _____

3. A 7-year-old child was evaluated for potential hearing loss. The child received a pure tone screening examination. Code for the service. _____
   _____

4. A patient with pneumonia received a penicillin injection IM. Code for the injection. _____
   _____

5. Code for the intramuscular administration of the human rabies immune globulin. _____
   _____

6. Code for the examination of the complete visual system for a new patient with determination of the refractive state. _____
   _____

7. A motor vehicle accident (MVA) leaves a patient with severe skin abrasions requiring debridement. The patient is sent to a wound care clinic and the nurse uses forceps and high pressure waterjet to debride a 15 sq. cm area. Code for the service. _____
   _____

8. Code for a transesophageal echocardiogram performed at the time of a cardiac surgery to monitor the patient's condition during surgery. _____
   _____

9. The patient received an IV infusion for therapeutic purposes for 1 hour. Code for the service. _____
   _____

10. A patient brings his allergy medication in a single dose vial to his internal medicine physician to receive a single injection. How will the internal medicine physician report this service? _____
    _____

CASE STUDIES

1. Mary R.

   Mary reported to her physician office to obtain vaccinations because she was going to South America on a mission trip. She received two injections for the yellow fever and typhoid (H-P) vaccines. The nurse had observed Mary for 5 minutes post-injection when she suddenly went into cardiac arrest. CPR was administered for 10 minutes until the ambulance arrived.

   Code for the vaccination services and CPR. _____

2. Grace M.

   Grace, a 62-year-old patient, is seen in the outpatient hemodialysis clinic three times a week for treatment of end-stage renal disease. She missed 7 days of therapy this month because of her vacation in Florida, but had one face-to-face visit with the physician during the month. A complete assessment had not been done this month.

   Assign the correct code to reflect services performed during the month. _____

3. Robert O.

   A physician orders a cardiovascular stress test on Robert, a 57-year-old male with recent ECG changes. Because Robert has a bad back and cannot walk fast enough on the treadmill without being fatigued, the physician orders a pharmacological stress test. An IV is started and dobutamine is given as a continuous drip with a gradual increase in the rate (at 3-minute intervals). Robert's heart rate accelerates, and an isotope is given when 85% of the target heart rate is achieved. A drop in the diastolic (lower number) blood pressure is generally awaited before administration of the isotope. Robert is asked to walk on the treadmill for a minute after the injection of isotope dipyridamole. The physician only supervises the test.

   Assign the procedure codes for the physician. _____

4. Arturo D.

   Percutaneous coronary intervention angioplasty of two branches of the left anterior descending artery was performed, followed by placement of a stent into both branches. An additional angioplasty was performed in the right coronary artery.

   Assign the procedure codes for these services. _____

5. Jerel A.

   Jerel, a 72-year-old woman, undergoes catheter placement in the coronary arteries with catheter placement into a left internal mammary artery bypass graft. Imaging supervision and interpretation were also provided.

   Assign the procedure codes for these services. _____

6. Samuel P.

   Samuel, a patient with a suspected embolism, sees his cardiologist who admits him to place a percutaneous catheter into the femoral artery of the left leg to perform thrombolysis. The catheter is advanced into the coronary artery, confirming the presence of an embolism in the artery. Intracoronary infusion is used to infuse the thrombolytic Eminase into the artery to dissolve the clot.

   Assign the procedure codes for the physician. _____

7. Marianna B.

   The physician provided the supervision and interpretation for a complete bilateral transcranial Doppler study of the intracranial arteries performed in the hospital. A copy of the analysis was placed in Marianna's medical record.

   Assign the procedure codes for the physician. _____

8. Christopher W.

Christopher, an 8-year-old patient, has severe ear pain. This has been a chronic problem for Christopher for the last 2 years. He also has a high fever. His mother calls the office at 8 p.m. even though the office has closed. The answering service reaches the pediatrician and he agrees to meet the boy and his mother at the office in an hour.

What CPT from the Medicine section should be reported in addition to the E/M service? _____

9. Shirley V.

Shirley, a 49-year-old patient, is being seen for her chemotherapy infusion. Because this patient has had significant problems with nausea and vomiting during previous episodes of chemotherapy, she will also receive a concurrent infusion of an antiemetic. The infusion lasts for 2 hours.

Assign the procedure codes for these services. _____

10. Zane Y.

Zane, a 24-year-old patient who experienced a catastrophic event in the workplace, meets with a psychiatrist for 45 minutes about his fears related to going back to work.

Code for the psychotherapy service. _____

INTERNET RESEARCH

Visit the Kidney Disease page at the American Kidney Foundation's website fat: www.kidneyfund .org/kidney-disease/ Click on "Kidney Failure/ESRD" and read the information. How is ERSD different from chronic kidney disease:

MEDICAL CODING LAB Remember to use the coding activities at **Medicalcodinglab.com** for extra practice on what you have just learned and to test your knowledge.

CHAPTER 30

HCPCS

The Healthcare Common Procedure Coding System (HCPCS) provides the national codes for medical products, supplies, and those services not included in CPT. These HCPCS codes are assigned along with a CPT code. Chapter 30 of *Conquer Medical Coding* explains the format of the system and the hierarchy for assigning the codes. In addition, the chapter explains the following topics:

- The circumstances under which codes from both HCPCS Level I and HCPCS Level II are required
- The difference between the permanent and temporary HCPCS codes
- The content and organization of the Index, Table of Drugs, and main text in HCPCS
- The sources of information needed to keep current with HCPCS changes
- The purpose and correct usage of HCPCS modifiers, including ABN modifiers
- How to choose the correct medication code based on the route of administration and the amount of medication administered
- The rules for choosing which level of HCPCS code to assign

CODE IT!

Supply the correct HCPCS codes for the following.

1. _____ Ocular implant

2. _____ Interphalangeal joint replacement

3. _____ Arthroscopic thermal capsulorrhaphy, left shoulder

4. _____ Arthroscopy of the knee with harvesting of cartilage (chondrocyte cells) for a Medicare patient

5. _____ Urethral stent (urolume)

6. _____ Implantable neurostimulator electrodes, per group of four

7. _____ Injection 0.5 mg digoxin

8. _____ Apnea monitor with recording, high-risk infant

9. _____ Adult hand prosthesis, mechanical, voluntary closing

10. _____ Sterile gloves, one pair

MULTIPLE CHOICE

Select the option that best completes the statement, or answers the question.

1. What is the correct HCPCS code assigned for parenteral nutrition supply kit, home mix?
   A. B4216
   B. B4220
   C. B4222
   D. B4224

2. What is the correct HCPCS code assigned for one tracheostomy mask?
   A. A7523
   B. A7524
   C. A7525
   D. A7526

3. What is the correct HCPCS code assigned for a wheelchair commode seat?
   A. E0968
   B. E0969
   C. E0970
   D. E9071

4. An outpatient alcohol crisis intervention is assigned which code?
   A. H0001
   B. H0004
   C. H0006
   D. H0007

5. What is the correct HCPCS code assigned for a replacement of a lithium battery for an external infusion pump that is owned by the patient?
   A. K0601
   B. K0602
   C. K0603
   D. K0604

6. An antireflective lens coating for two lenses is coded as:
   A. V2750
   B. V2750 × 2
   C. V2755
   D. V2755 × 2

7. A patient is seen in the OB/GYN office for insertion of a Skyla IUD for birth control. The provider would report which codes?
   A. 58300, J7306
   B. 58300, J7297
   C. 58300, J7300
   D. 58300, J7301

8. A patient is seen in the emergency department (ED) with acute on chronic angina. The physician orders a myocardial profusion study with Technetium TC 99m sestamibi. What is the correct way to code this situation?
   A. A9520
   B. A9510
   C. A9500
   D. A9502

9. A patient with breast cancer is admitted for mastectomy with immediate reconstruction with breast implant. Assign the code for the implant.
   A. L8600
   B. L8000
   C. L8010
   D. L8020

10. A patient suffers chemical burns of the forearm. The physician debrides the skin and performs skin replacement surgery, placing 10 sq. cm of Apligraf. What is the correct way to code this situation?
    A. Q4106
    B. Q4100
    C. Q4101
    D. Q4101 × 5

SHORT ANSWER

Answer the following questions.

For questions 1 to 3, look up the code. Identify the notation(s) that appears for each code. Look at the color coding and symbols to determine if information on coverage is supplied. If so, list it as well.

Notation(s)/Coverage

1. A4206 *Syringe with needle, sterile 1 cc, 1 each* _____

2. A4550 *Surgical trays* _____

3. J2995 *Injection, Streptokinase, per 250,000 IU* _____

4. A patient was seen in the ED with acute agitation. The patient received an initial dose of 3 mg of Lorazepam IM. Thirty minutes later, the patient received another 3 mg to control agitation and maintain a desired level of sedation. Fill in the following information based on the scenario.

HCPCS Code	OPPS Status	Units
_____	_____	_____

   Will the facility receive a separate payment for this drug? Why or why not? _____

   _____

5. Determining a patient's insurance information will help the coder decide whether a HCPCS level or Level II code is needed. Why is this? _____

   _____

   _____

6. When a provider is level-setting practice fees against the costs for services and supplies in the practice, where does the provider go to determine the allowed amount for drugs commonly administered in the office, considering they do not reside on the MPFS? _____

_____

7. Research modifier AU and explain why it is used and with which codes. This modifier is appended to HCPCS codes but it is also an abbreviation that means what? _____

_____

_____

8. A perimenopausal woman is seen in the GYN office for complaints of hot flashes, fatigue, decreased libido, and weight gain. The physician places one estrogen and one testosterone pellet subcutaneously in her right hip. What are the HCPCS codes for the implants? Research Medicare coverage policies and explain if this service is a covered benefit. _____

_____

_____

9. Patients with prescriptions for home oxygen require equipment to store and transport the tanks as well as concentrators, regulators, and battery packs for use at home. Equipment is rented on a monthly basis. What is the code for renting a portable oxygen system for home use? What is included in this code? What does the indicated Medicare coverage policy say about this code and how it should be reported to indicate it is being rented? _____

_____

_____

_____

10. Find the code for a semi-electric hospital bed with mattress. What does the Medicare coverage limitations say about reporting hospital beds and which modifiers should be submitted? _____

_____

_____

_____

CASE STUDIES

1. Colleen A.

   Colleen, a patient with colon cancer, is admitted for colectomy with a colostomy drainable pouch for use on a barrier with a locking flange with filter.

   What HCPCS code will the facility report for the colostomy device? _____

2. Alexia O.

   Alexia is admitted for total knee replacement due to severe osteoarthritis. The physician inserted a bicompartmental joint implant.

   What HCPCS code will the facility report? _____

3. Joel Y.

Joel had a syncopal event and presented to the ED via ambulance. EKG was positive for a third-degree heart block. He required dual-chamber rate responsive pacemaker insertion with transvenous lead insertion into the atrium and ventricle.

Assign the HCPCS code for the pacemaker. _____

4. Deidra V.

Deidra fell out of her wheelchair at the nursing home. Upon evaluation, she complained of headache, blurred vision, and pain in her left leg. She was diagnosed with a concussion and nondisplaced fracture of the tibial shaft. Her treatment was complicated by her multiple sclerosis. The fracture was treated by fiberglass air cast application.

Assign the HCPCS code for the air cast. _____

5. Fuhua M.

Fuhua came to the hospital because of flank pain and hematuria. Cystoscopy with retro-grade pyelogram was positive for ureteral calculus and hydronephrosis. Later, he underwent cystourethroscopy with basket extraction of ureteral calculus and insertion of indwelling ureteral stent.

Assign the HCPCS code for the indwelling stent. _____

6. Chilo H.

Chilo had his tonsils taken out 2 days ago. He now presents with postoperative hemorrhage status post tonsillectomy. He requires control of his bleeding and was given Demerol 95 mg IM for pain.

Assign the HCPCS code for the Demerol. _____

7. Harry S.

Harry, a chemotherapy patient suffering from anemia secondary to treatment, presents to his oncologist's office for his routine B_{12} injection for vitamin B_{12} deficiency anemia due to chemotherapy. Sytobex 1000 mg IM was provided.

Assign the HCPCS code for the Sytobex. _____

8. JoBeth S.

JoBeth, a diabetic patient, sees her podiatrist for her quarterly foot check and nail trim. Her nails are very thick with onychomycosis. The physician uses a motorized shaver and trimmers to cut all 10 nails.

Assign the HCPCS code for the nail trimming. _____

9. Shantel E.

Shantel, a 4-day-old newborn delivered by cesarean section, is in the neonatal intensive care unit (NICU) and is being followed by the NICU attending for her continued tachypnea and jaundice. She has been placed on continued positive airway pressure (CPAP) in order to control the tachypnea.

Assign the HCPCS code for the CPAP. _____

10. Brittney L.

Brittney presented to the ED with headaches. CT of the brain without contrast was nega-tive. Her headaches were due to migraines as documented by the ED physician. Toradol 15 mg IV was administered before leaving the ED.

Assign the HCPCS code for the Toradol. _____

INTERNET RESEARCH

1. Visit the CMS website listed here and report on the most current HCPCS quarterly updates. Include any new temporary codes that will go into effect. www.cms.gov/HCPCSRelease-CodeSets/https://www.cms.gov/Medicare/Coding/HCPCSReleaseCodeSets/HCPCS-Quarterly-Update.html
2. Visit carrier websites such as Aetna, Blue Cross/Blue Shield, or United Healthcare and read about their payment and reporting policies for HCPCS. Write a brief report of your findings. www.aetna.com and www.bcbsm.com
3. Determine which DME MAC you would report DME claims to based on the geographic location of your patient. Search the carrier's website for NCD or LCD policies pertaining to E0601. Which criteria must be met to bill this code?
4. Visit the CMS website and search for the MUE for code L0120. What is the MUE value for this supply?

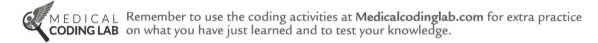 Remember to use the coding activities at **Medicalcodinglab.com** for extra practice on what you have just learned and to test your knowledge.

Answers

CHAPTER 1 Your Career as a Medical Coder

Multiple Choice

1. b
2. b, c, d
3. b
4. b, d
5. a
6. b
7. d
8. b
9. a, b, d
10. b

Short Answer

1. Encounter form, superbill
2. Outpatient
3. Subjective
4. Diagnoses
5. ICD-10-CM
6. ICD-10-PCS
7. Self-funded health plans
8. Operational

9. Outpatient clinics and ASCs

10. Patient's medical record

11. CPC

12. Hospital

13. AHIMA

14. EMTALA

15. Medical coding

16. ICD-10-PCS

17. Revenue cycle

18. Medicare

19. Health insurance company, computer system vendors

20. Same-day procedures, screening examinations

Case Studies

1. Yes, EMTALA

2. No. She is not likely to be hired because communication skills, both written and verbal, are as important as knowing about how to code for medical services.

3. No, many years of experience can lead to many years of incorrect coding information passed down from one coder to another. A coding certification demonstrates a superior level of skill by passing a written proficiency test.

4. No, the procedure would be considered cosmetic, and would not be covered by health insurance.

5. No, CHAMPVA covers veterans and their dependents, including the dependents of veterans who died from service-related disabilities.

6. Ingrown toenails, to trim and soak his nails and to change his footwear.

7. Yes, she was treated with nitroglycerin and instructed to see her cardiologist as soon as possible.

8. Warts, CO_2 laser

9. No, a tee shirt and jeans are not appropriate in a professional setting. In preparing for an interview, an applicant should leave adequate time for unforeseen circumstances. The applicant's attire and lateness would make him a poor candidate for a coding position.

10. She is describing a billing position and most likely would not be hired because of her attitude toward IT issues. She needed to be more positive in regard to computer programs for medical billing and to talk about her coding skills, not her billing responsibilities from a time that is no longer relevant in physician practices.

CHAPTER 2 The Regulatory Environment of Coding

Multiple Choice

1. a, b, c

2. b

3. c

4. a, c, d

5. c

6. a

7. b

8. b

9. c

10. a

Short Answer

1. Presenting problem

2. Informed consent

3. Discharge summary

4. Documentation

5. Office of the Inspector General (OIG)

6. Fraud

7. No

8. Affordable Care Act

9. Standard transactions

10. Centers for Medicare and Medicaid

11. Joint Commission on Accreditation of Healthcare Organizations (JCAHO)

12. Rescission

13. No, whether a code will be reimbursed depends on whether it has been correctly coded. Some codes are included in the payment for other codes based on CPT coding guidelines.

14. Office of the Inspector General

15. Physician training and staff training

16. No, it is most often documented in the patient's own words.

17. Physical examination and diagnosis

18. Progress note

19. A complete history and physical (H&P) is documented with four types of information: (1) the chief complaint, (2) the history and physical examination, (3) the diagnosis or assessment, and (4) the treatment plan.

20. Conditions of participation

Case Studies

1. No, the patient's health information (PHI) may be disclosed for purposes of treatment, payment, and health-care operations (TPO).

2. No, changing the date of service of the patient's encounter is considered fraud.

3. Bilateral lower extremity swelling and shortness of breath

4. Removal of nasal tumor, pathology

5. Yes, this is a breach of protected health information (PHI).

6. No, HCPCS codes are one of the three code sets required under HIPAA.

7. The coder: The type of services provided that day specifically describes the codes for discharge day management.

8. No, Parkinson's disease has not been determined; the physician specifically indicated that he was questioning whether or not the patient had that disease. The correct diagnosis for that visit is the symptoms the patient presented with: headaches, abnormal gait.

9. Examination

10. Immediate access to health information

CHAPTER 3 ICD-10-CM Basics

Code It!

1. J01.01

2. J35.3

3. A22.1

4. E11.41, Z79.4

5. E04.2

6. E27.1

7. C50.512

8. J96.01, C34.31

9. T74.12XA

10. S82.252

Multiple Choice

1. d

2. c

3. d (abnormal liver function tests not integral to both; therefore, code the sign separately)

4. c

5. d

6. a

7. b

8. a

9. a

10. d

Short Answer

1. Current code books and updated computer systems

2. October 1st

3. The letter X

4. No, the coder must verify the code in the ICD-10-CM Tabular List to obtain the correct code and read all the associated notes and instructions.

5. Excludes2 note

6. and/or

7. Tabular List

8. Sequelae

9. Index to External Causes of Injury

10. HIPAA legislation

Case Studies

1. a. Lymphadenopathy. b. R59.0.

2. a. Frequency, nocturia. b. R35.0, R35.1.

3. a. Elevated. b. R03.0, R12.

4. a. Right lower quadrant. b. R10.31, N89.8.

5. a. Use additional code (B95–B97) to identify infectious agent. b. Block L00–L08. c. Abbreviation Book. d. L03.116, B95.62, E10.9.

6. a. Syncope. b. Syndrome. c. I49.5, G89.29, M54.9.

7. a. Anatomy Book. b. See Derangement knee, meniscus, caused by old tear. c. M94.262, M23.252, M12.262.

8. a. Yes. b. R94.5, F10.10, I10.

9. a. An autoimmune disease of blood vessels. b. Medical dictionary. c. M30.3.

10. a. Table of Drugs and Chemicals. b. Congestive heart failure. c. N39.0, I50.43, T50.1X6A.

CHAPTER 4 ICD-10-CM Coding Guidelines

Code It!

1. I25.110

2. I11.0, I50.9

3. I63.40, I69.359

4. I70.245, I03.116

5. T82.7XXA, L03.115

6. M05.10

7. B20, C46.0

8. T63.441A

9. D50.9, D59.9

10. 10 I88.0, D68.4

Multiple Choice

1. d

2. c

3. a

4. a

5. d

6. d

7. a

8. c

9. c

10. a

Short Answer

1. That condition established after study to be chiefly responsible for occasioning the admission of the patient to the hospital for care.

2. Clinical evaluation; or therapeutic treatment; or diagnostic procedures; or extended length of hospital stay; or increased nursing care or monitoring

3. When the condition develops after admission

4. MS-DRGs

5. The complication

6. Versus, Or

7. Operative report

8. Discharge summary or discharge record

9. Physician orders

10. Conditions documented as "ruled out" should not be reported; conditions documented as "rule out" at discharge should be reported.

Case Studies

1. a. No. b. E11.51, E11.621, L97.529, E11.21, E11.622, L97.229.

2. a. Examination. b. K57.32.

3. a. High-density lipoprotein. b. E11.9, I25.10.

4. a. Right arm pain. b. Yes, sickle cell anemia. c. Z88.8.

5. a. Suprapubic pain, difficulty urinating. b. N40.1, R33.8.

6. a. Yes, coronary artery disease, history of myocardial infarction, status post pacemaker. b. R04.0, I11.9, I25.10, I25.2, Z95.0.

7. a. No. b. R07.89, M79.631.

8. a. Left knee swelling. b. Acute bursitis of the knee. c. M25.462, F17.210, J45.41.

9. a. Acute hypoxic respiratory failure. b. J96.01.

10. a. Acute and chronic conditions, Section I.B.8. b. K85.9, K86.1, K70.30, F19.21, Z85.46.

CHAPTER 5 ICD-10-CM Chapters 1 Through 5: A00–F99

Code It!

1. A02.0

2. B37.2

3. L02.212, B95.62

4. C40.22, M89.762

5. D57.01

6. C18.4, D63.0

7. E10.622, L97.51

8. A41.01, R65.21

9. E43, Z68.1

10. F13.282, F14.11

Multiple Choice

1. a

2. a

3. c

4. d

5. a

6. d

7. c

8. b

9. c

10. c

Short Answer

1. Pharmacokinetics

2. Oseltamivir

3. Ovary

4. Leukocytosis, fever, tachypnea or tachycardia (two of these)

5. Contiguous sites

6. Physician query

7. Stimulate the production of red blood cells

8. Gestational diabetes

9. Obese (severe)

10. *DSM-V (Diagnostic and Statistical Manual of Mental Disorders*–5th Edition)

Case Studies

1. a. No (integral to acute pancreatitis). b. Acute pancreatitis. c. K85.2, K86.0, F10.20, Z71.41 (counseling).

2. a. True. b. C47.3.

3. a. Symptoms of fatigue, low hemoglobin and hematocrit. b. Aplastic anemia. c. True. d. D61.1, C18.7, C78.7, T45.1x5A.

4. a. Urinary tract. b. No. c. Yes (with organ dysfunction). d. A41.5, R65.20, N17.9, N39.0.

5. a. Yes. b. Accidental poisoning. c. Nephropathy and neuropathy. d. Hypoglycemia. e. T85.614A, T38.3x1A, E10.649, E10.21, E10.40.

6. a. Yes. b. F14.23, F10.231, F17.210, K70.30, F20.0.

7. a. Section 1.C, Chapter 2, Section e.3. b. Z51.0. c. C50.512, E66.01, Z68.43.

8. a. Dysuria and flank pain. b. Methicillin-resistant *Staphylococcus aureus*. c. Acute. d. N30.00, N30.20, B95.62, E87.6, E83.42.

9. E11.52, Z79.4

10. a. No. b. AIDS/HIV disease. c. B20, B59, F11.90.

CHAPTER 6 ICD-10-CM Chapters 6 Through 10: G00–J99

Code It!

1. I50.33
2. I13.10, N18.4
3. J45.90, J44.9
4. J01.80, B95.62
5. H35.033, I10
6. H90.3
7. H70.11
8. G44.011
9. G31.83, F02.80
10. I71.4

Multiple Choice

1. a
2. b
3. d
4. a
5. b
6. a
7. b
8. c
9. a
10. d

Short Answer

1. Four (4) weeks
2. Chest pain
3. Yes (GI bleed is caused by gastritis)
4. CKD and heart disease classified to I50.- and I51.4–I51.9
5. Blindness categories 3, 4, and 5
6. When the reason for the encounter is pain control and not treatment of the underlying condition
7. Chronic asthmatic (obstructive) bronchitis, chronic bronchitis with emphysema or airway obstruction, chronic obstructive asthma, bronchitis, or tracheobronchitis

8. It is a worsening or decompensation of a chronic condition.

9. General

10. Nondominant

Case Studies

1. a. Malaise, fever, cough. b. J20.9.

2. R04.2, R06.02, F17.210

3. a. Cardiac catheterization. b. I25.110, E11.9, E78.2.

4. a. Code first. b. T55.1X1A, H10.213.

5. G44.201, H53.142

6. J21.19

7. a. Epistaxis. b. R04.0, J44.9, M15.9, Z87.891, Z99.81.

8. a. Section I.C.6.b.1.a (Chapter Guidelines, Chapter 6 Section b.1.a). b. G89.29, M51.26.

9. a. Facial droop, dysphasia, left hemiplegia. b. I63.532, R29.810, R47.02, G81.02, I10, I48.2, Z79.01.

10. a. Tachycardia–bradycardia syndrome. b. I49.5, I21.A9.

CHAPTER 7 ICD-10-CM Chapters 11 Through 14: K00–N99

Code It!

1. A04.71

2. K72.00, K74.60

3. K57.32, K65.9

4. K85.1, K80.00

5. N80.0

6. L20.84

7. L23.7

8. M06.00

9. N39.41, R35.0

10. M20.1, M20.41

Multiple Choice

1. c

2. a

3. b

4. c

5. b

6. d

7. a

8. d

9. c

10. b

Short Answer

1. Low hemoglobin and hematocrit

2. Ringworm

3. Stage III (3)

4. Right upper extremity

5. Total abdominal hysterectomy

6. Opioid

7. Stage II (2)

8. Adverse reaction

9. Anticholinergics

10. Lower urinary tract symptoms

Case Studies

1. L70.0, L73.0

2. a. Urinary frequency, periumbilical abdominal pain. b. N34.2.

3. N30.00, I11.9

4. M17.12, M1A.00, E11.9

5. a. Old cerebral infarction with right hemiplegia and aphasia. b. K26.0, D62, I69.351, I69.320.

6. a. See Calculus bile duct. b. K80.42, Z53.31. (code also the procedure converted from laparoscopic to open)

7. a. Large intestine. b. K50.812, K50.811.

8. D25.2, D27.1, D50.0

9. N84.0

10. C67.8

CHAPTER 8 ICD-10-CM Chapters 15 Through 17: O00–Q99

Code It!

1. Z39.2

2. P55.1

3. Z05.1

4. Z38.01, P04.49

5. Q25.71

6. O24.012, Z3A.22, E11.10

7. O62.1, O76, Z37.0, Z3A.37

8. O30.043, O66.5, Z37.2, Z3A.38

9. J18.9, P78.83

10. Z37.3

Multiple Choice

1. c

2. a

3. d

4. b

5. a

6. b

7. d

8. a

9. b

10. b

Short Answer

1. Caffeine

2. Surfactant

3. Tocolytics

4. Spontaneous abortion

5. Six (6) weeks

6. In childbirth

7. Third trimester

8. Zero (0)

9. No, a twin pregnancy is not a normal pregnancy.

10. N

Case Studies

1. a. O09.513, O60.14x0, O44.03, Z3A.35, Z37.0. b. Z38.00, P07.38, P07.17.

2. a. O60.14, O76, Z37.2, Z3A.36. b. Z38.31, P29.12, P07.39, P07.18. c. Z38.31, P07.39, P07.18.

3. O60.03, Z87.51

4. a. O48.0, O34.21, O36.63, Z87.51, Z37.0. b. Z38.01, P08.1.

5. Z00.110, P07.35, P07.16

6. O03.5, B95.61

7. a. O14.13, O13.3, O76, O60.14x0, O90.8, Z3A.34, Z37.0. b. Z38.01, P07.37, P29.12.

8. a. O80, Z37.0, Z30.2, Z3A.39. b. Z38.00.

9. a. O24.02, O30.103, O99.824, Z3A.38, Z37.51. b. Z38.6x3.

10. Z38.31, P36.4, P28.4, P05.08

CHAPTER 9 ICD-10-CM Chapters 18 Through 21: R00–Z99

Code It!

1. Z12.11, K57.32
2. Z51.0, C79.51, Z85.46
3. Z23
4. T86.11, N17.9
5. T22.332A, T31.0, X17.XXXA, Y92.63
6. J44.1, Z99.11
7. K92.2, T45.515A
8. Z03.71
9. T84.041A
10. J95.830, Y83.6

Multiple Choice

1. a
2. b
3. d
4. a
5. b
6. b
7. c
8. d
9. a
10. b

Short Answer

1. Displaced
2. No, a causal relationship is not documented between the current infection and catheter.
3. 18%
4. Acetaminophen
5. Acute exacerbation of asthma
6. Poisoning
7. Motor response, opening of eyes, and verbal response
8. D (routine healing)
9. Yes
10. Activity

Case Studies

1. a. Y83.6. b. Z40.01, Z80.2, T81.4XXA, B95.61, Y83.6.
2. a. Accident. b. S02.0XXA, S06.2X5A, S27.321A, S36.114A, V86.55XA.

3. a. Y92.039. b. Poisoning. c. T40.5X1A, T51.91XA, T42.3X1A, R40.244.

4. a. K91.89. b. K56.69, L76.22, Y83.2.

5. a. Adverse reaction. b. Sigmoid colon. c. E86.0, D70.1, C18.7, C78.7, T45.1X5A, T80.90XA, I50.9.

6. a. External cause of injury codes for mechanism and place of injury; loss of consciousness. b. S02.119A, S06.5X0A.

7. a. Superficial bites. b. S61.451A, S61.350A, S63.264A, W54.0XXA, Y92.017A.

8. a. R40.2132, R40.2242, R40.2362. b. W212.20A, Y92.330, Y93.22. c. As associated head wound (S01.–) or skull fracture (S02.–). d. S06.0X1A.

9. a. Chronic kidney disease. b. Yes. c. N18.6, Z99.2, Z76.82, T82.7XXA, L03.114, Y83.1.

10. a. Shortness of breath, wheezing, itching. b. Yes. c. D. d. J44.1, S51.811D, Z91.120, T48.6X6A, T36.0X5A, L29.8, W26.0XXD.

CHAPTER 10 ICD-10-CM Outpatient Coding Guidelines

Code It!

1. R10.31

2. L55.1

3. I83.024, L97.423

4. K92.1, Z80.0

5. J10.10

6. I69.821

7. Z02.89

8. J44.1, E10.9

9. M25.572

10. K81.1, G89.18

Multiple Choice

1. c

2. a

3. b

4. a

5. d

6. c

7. b

8. a

9. d

10. b

Short Answer

1. Outpatient

2. Inguinal hernia

3. Yes

4. First listed diagnosis

5. Principal diagnosis

6. Yes

7. Weakness, fever, flank pain

8. Screening colonoscopy

9. O09.512

10. Section IV. Paragraph J

Case Studies

1. I10, I48.2, J44.9, Z23

2. a. Z01.818. b. M23.200, E10.40.

3. F10.129, Y90.5, E87.1

4. F11.10, M54.5, G89.29

5. a. Section IV.A.2. b. Z12.11, D12.5, I95.81.

6. a. Passed out. b. E09.649, T38.0x5A, M06.9.

7. J35.01, J95.830

8. I50.23, T50.1X6a, Z91.120

9. a. Chronic Kidney Disease. b. N13.1.

10. a. M25.572. b. S82.842A. c. S82.842A. d. W09.1XXA, Y92.830. e. S82.842D.

CHAPTER 11 ICD-10-PCS Overview and Format

Code It!

1. 0Y913ZZ

2. 0FT44ZZ

3. 0B9P3ZX

4. 0TY00Z0

5. 0SRC0J9

6. B41G1ZZ

7. DB0Z3ZZ

8. F06Z8KZ

9. 10D00Z1

10. 0CJS8ZZ

Multiple Choice

1. d

2. a

3. a

4. b

5. d

6. b

7. a

8. d

9. c

10. c

Short Answer

1. Never

2. Release

3. One

4. CPT

5. Should not

6. Irrigation

7. Diaphragm

8. Percutaneous endoscopic

9. Administration

10. Measurement

Case Studies

1. Excision, 0DBN8ZZ

2. Via natural or artificial opening endoscopic, 0TJB8ZZ

3. Percutaneous, 0VB03ZX

4. Extraluminal, 0UL74CZ

5. Lower, 0ST20ZZ

6. Extraocular, 08SM0ZZ

7. One, 0HBU0ZX

8. K-Wire, 0PSP04Z

9. No, 027034Z

10. 0CTQXZZ, 0CTPXZZ (either order)

CHAPTER 12 CPT Basics

Code It!

1. 19100

2. 20526

3. 20250

4. 46030

5. 96999

6. 47579

7. 47

8. 22

9. RT, T8

10. 62

Multiple Choice

1. a

2. c

3. c

4. d

5. d

6. b

7. d

8. a

9. d

10. b

Short Answer

1. 47, 23

2. Unlisted procedure, add-on codes, ⊘ modifier –51 exempt codes

3. AMA

4. 53

5. October 1, January 1 the following year

6. Add-on

7. –51

8. Performed alone, a separate site, during a separate session

9. Procedure, condition, abbreviation, eponym, body site, symptom

10. a. Heading. b. Section. c. Subcategory. d. Procedure. e. Subsection.

Case Studies

1. 55

2. Yes, parenthetical instructions located at the end of the colposcopy of cervix section say, "For endometrial sampling (biopsy) performed in conjunction with colposcopy, use 58110." When the coder refers to code 58110, it is noted that this is an add-on code and another parenthetical note instructs the coder to report 58110 in addition to 57452–57461.

3. 19105-RT, 19105-RT-59. Two codes are reported because the probe was inserted twice.

4. 56

5. a. Venipuncture and steroid injection. These are not add-on codes and not part of the E/M office visit and can be billed independently. b. 36415, 96372. c. Yes, 99213–25. The –25 modifier is only reported on the E/M code. Some payers may bundle 36415 into the office

visit as part of their payment policy; however, from a coding guideline perspective, it can be reported separately.

6. a. 20 urgent care. b. Chest x-ray, nebulizer, IV steroid administration. c. 71046-TC, 94640, 96374.

7. a. 23. b. 93880, 93000. The facility reports the complete EKG code because the tracing and interpretation were performed in the emergency department.

8. 5005F, 2029F

9. a. 58565. b. Reduced service. Parenthetical notes tell the coder to report modifier –52 for unilateral procedures. c. –52. d. Yes, the anesthetist.

10. a. Annually. b. Annually. Category II and III codes and vaccine codes are updated twice a year on January 1st and July 1st. Each October codes are released but do not take effect until January 1. c. The AMA website publishes changes each quarter. CPT manual Appendices B, E, F, K, and N.

CHAPTER 13 CPT: Evaluation and Management Codes

Code It!

1. 99466

2. Observation care 99218

3. 99213

4. 99468. Do not use the critical care codes 99291, 99292 when the neonate is inpatient. The inpatient codes are per-day codes and time is not a factor.

5. 99374. Care plan oversight

6. 99203

7. 99284

8. 99252. For new patient the code can be no higher than the lowest key component.

9. 99201–99205. This is a new patient service.

10. Care plan oversight services 99378

Multiple Choice

1. a

2. b

3. a

4. d

5. a

6. c

7. a

8. b

9. c

10. a

Short Answer

1. When more than 50% of the total visit time is based on counseling and/or coordination of care

2. The roll-up rule applies when more than one E/M service is provided on the same date by the same physician for the same patient. When that occurs, all services will roll up into the greater E/M service. (Note that there are exceptions to the roll-up rule.)

3. Rarely do all three key components match the requirements of the E/M code descriptors. When one of the key components is at a lower level of service, it controls the code to be reported. Keep in mind which codes require all three key components versus two of three key components.

4. The physician is incorrect. CPT does provide for that situation. Report code 99358, which specifically provides for this prolonged E/M service "before and/or after direct patient care."

5. Codes 99339–99340 are for services to patients who are either at home or in a domiciliary residence and are not under the care of a home health agency, hospice, or nursing facility. Codes 99374–99380 are specific to patients under the care of a home health agency, hospice, or nursing facility.

6. The statement does not represent an established concept; the concept is a myth. This is a common misconception about consultation services and is clearly addressed in this chapter and the CPT book consultation guidelines. A consultant is allowed to provide treatment during a consultation service.

7. The 15-minute rule means that you can report the add-on code once you have passed 14 minutes beyond the time represented in the parent code. Pediatric critical care transport codes: 99466–99486; critical care codes: 99291–99292; prolonged physician services: 99354–99359.

8. 99215, 99354

9. 99231–99233

10. 99471

Case Studies

1. The coder is not correct. As indicated early on in this chapter, an E/M level of service is determined by the three key components of history, examination, and medical decision making. The contributory components do not affect the level of service.

2. Multiple diagnoses indicate moderate complexity, limited data indicates low complexity, and low risk is low complexity. Two of these three elements must be met or exceeded. The complexity is low.

3. The history was detailed 99203, examination was EPF 99202, and the MDM was low 99203. New patient codes require that all three key components must meet or exceed the level of service reported. That means the lowest key component 99202 controls the level of service.

4. 99291, 99292x2

5. 99252

6. 99396, 99213–25

7. In an established patient visit, only two of the three key components are required. The lower of the three key components is dropped and the encounter is based on the remaining two. A detailed history and moderate medical decision making are coded as 99214.

8. Although the case study emphasizes the time spent during the visit, the rule for using time as the determining factor for the level of service has not been met. Greater than 50% of the total visit time must be spent in counseling to use time. The key components are PF history 99212, EPF examination 99213, and low MDM 99213. In an established patient visit,

only two of the three key components are required. The history level dropped and the code is 99213.

9. Consultations are based on all three key components. The code can be no higher than 99253 regardless of the level of MDM.

10. This is not a follow-up consultation, so the correct code for these services is subsequent hospital care 99231.

CHAPTER 14 CPT: Evaluation and Management Auditing

Code It!

1. Brief

2. Extended

3. Complete

4. EPF, 99202

5. EPF, 99202

6. Moderate

7. Minimal

8. Low

9. Low

10. 99202

Multiple Choice

1. a. First, always check at the end of the question to verify what the question is asking. Review of the information shows at least four HPI = extended = detailed, five ROS = extended = detailed, one PFSH for an established patient = pertinent. All components of history are at the same level—detailed.

2. b. In review of the answers, a is an office or outpatient consult, whereas b–d are hospital consult codes. A quick review of the question shows that this is a hospital consultation, which eliminates answer a. The history level is detailed as indicated in the question, which is code 99253. The MDM level is given as moderate, which is code 99254. The question shows that the cardiologist examined three organ systems, which is the EPF examination code 99252. A consultation code LOS requires all three key components to be at the LOS reported or choose the lowest key component of the three. The cardiologist must report code 99252.

3. c. Documentation of the abdominal pain is the diagnosis or management option component of MDM. Ordering blood work and barium swallow and review of the results is the amount and complexity of the data component of MDM. The possibility of scheduling surgery is the overall risk component of MDM.

4. a. Note that the question states this is an established patient. That eliminates c and d because 99203 is a new patient code and the documentation of only two key components is allowed for an established patient. For history, the physician documented a brief HPI based on location (abdomen), context (too many sweets), and her lethargy in a review of systems (ROS). The examination was EPF, based on the examination of the digestive system and the constitutional system. MDM was moderate based on the abdominal pain, which is new to the physician. The data review of the blood work and x-ray and the overall risk is given as moderate. When these elements are placed into the audit form, you will have an EPF history and examination and moderate MDM. The LOS can be no higher than the lowest key component, which is the EPF level. That LOS is then code 99213.

5. b. History: Three HPI = brief, three systems reviewed = extended, past and family history = complete for an established patient. These three elements = an EPF history, which is code 99213.
   EXAMINATION: Three organ systems examined = an EPF examination, which is 99213.
   MDM: Low, which is 99213.
   The level of service is 99213.

6. b. An EPF history and examination with low MDM is 99202.

7. a. In the 1997 musculoskeletal examination guidelines, one to five elements identified by a bullet equals a PF level. The five bullets are constitutional, neck nodes, gait, asymmetry, and range of motion.

8. a. The LOS is the same; the general multisystem examination requirements are one to five elements identified by a bullet for a PF level.

9. c

10. b

Short Answer

1. The first set of guidelines (1995) did not meet the needs of many of the specialty physicians; the second set (1997) was created to meet those needs.

2. HPI, context

3. Yes

4. Both

5. History, review of systems

6. Review of systems

7. Documentation of two of the PFSH criteria is allowed as a complete level of PFSH for established patients and ED patients.

8. Yes

9. Yes

10. Overall risk

Case Studies

1. 99213.
   DETAILED HISTORY: 4 HPI, 2 ROS, 1 PFSH
   EPF examination: Eyes, ENT, respiratory, skin
   Low MDM: Established problem worsening, no data review, moderate overall risk based on prescription medication. Lowest key component(s) controls LOS.

2. 99214.
   DETAILED HISTORY: 4 HPI, 5 ROS, 3 PFSH
   EPF EXAMINATION: Constitutional, cardiovascular, gastrointestinal, respiratory
   MODERATE MDM: New problem with additional workup, no data review, moderate overall risk based on the EGD procedure. For an established patient, you need only two key components to determine the LOS; history and examination are both at the 99214 level.

3. a. Laceration on bridge of nose. b. Extended: Location—nose, quality—bleeding, severity—no loss of consciousness, context—fall. c. Extended: Cardiovascular, allergies. d. Pertinent: Documentation of medication. e. EPF: Constitutional, ENT, skin, neck. f. Low: New problem with no additional workup, no data review, low overall risk based on presenting problem of acute uncomplicated injury. g. 99282. Even though the history is detailed (99283), both the examination and MDM are at the 99282 level.

4. 99212.
   EPF HISTORY: 4 HPI, 1 ROS, no PFSH
   PF EXAMINATION: Eyes—1 bullet, arm—1 bullet, lungs—1 bullet, GI—2 bullets (total 5 bullets)
   LOW MDM: New problem, no additional workup, no data review, low overall risk based on acute uncomplicated injury.

5. New patient code is 99203.
   COMPREHENSIVE HISTORY: 4 HPI, 10+ ROS, all 3 PFSH
   DETAILED EXAMINATION: Constitutional, cardiovascular, eyes, GI, musculoskeletal, respiratory
   HIGH MDM: New problem, additional workup, extensive data review—laboratory tests and EKG ordered and independent visualization done of EKG, moderate overall risk based on presenting problem of undiagnosed new problem.
   For a new patient, the code can be no higher than the lowest key component of all three components documented. The lowest key component is the detailed examination and the code associated with a detailed examination is 99203 for a new patient.

6. E/M code is 99214.
   DETAILED HISTORY: 4 HPI, 2 ROS, 1 PFSH
   DETAILED EXAMINATION: Constitutional, ENT, respiratory, skin, lymphatic
   MODERATE MDM: New problem with no additional workup, x-ray ordered with independent visualization, moderate risk based on antibiotic prescription drug management.

7. E/M code is 99282.
   DETAILED HISTORY: 4 HPI, 2 ROS, 3 PFSH
   EPF EXAMINATION: Constitutional, neurological, skin
   LOW MDM: New problem with additional workup, no data review, low risk based on presenting problem and management options.

8. E/M code is 99202.
   EPF HISTORY: 2 HPI, 2 ROS, 2 PFSH
   EPF EXAMINATION: Eyes, skin, lymphatic, head
   LOW MDM: New problem with additional workup, no data review, low risk based on diagnostic procedures planned—skin biopsies.

9. E/M code is 99213.
   DETAILED HISTORY: 5 HPI, 2 ROS, 1 PFSH
   PF EXAMINATION: Skin
   LOW MDM: New problem with additional workup, no data review, low risk based on diagnostic procedures planned—laser ablation.
   NOTE: Detailed history = 99214, PF examination = 99212, low MDM = 99213. Drop the lowest key component (examination 99212) and base the LOS on the remaining two key components, select the lowest of the two.

10. E/M code is 99214.
    DETAILED HISTORY: 4 HPI, 3 ROS, 1 PFSH
    DETAILED EXAMINATION: Constitutional, cardiovascular, eyes, gastrointestinal, respiratory
    MODERATE MDM: New problem with additional workup, one data review for blood work, moderate risk based on presenting problem of undiagnosed new problem with uncertain prognosis.

CHAPTER 15 CPT: Anesthesia Codes

Code It!

1. 00454. Locate anesthesia, clavicle in the CPT Index.

2. 01961, QZ. Locate anesthesia, cesarean in the CPT Index. This procedure requires the QZ modifier to represent that the CRNA was not under the medical direction of the anesthesiologist.

3. 01400, AA. You will find this code most efficiently by reviewing the anesthesia section rather than the CPT Index. Find the header for the knee and choose the code that

represents surgical arthroscopy of the knee not otherwise specified. There are two other codes that are more specific, but neither of them is correct. The question specified the procedure was performed by the anesthesiologist, which requires the AA modifier.

4. 00914. You will find this code most efficiently by reviewing the anesthesia section rather than the CPT Index. Find the perineum header and review the code descriptions.

5. 00172. Locate anesthesia, cleft palate in the CPT Index.

6. 00160. You will find this code most efficiently by reviewing the anesthesia section rather than the CPT Index. This code is under the header for procedures on the nose and accessory sinuses not otherwise specified.

7. 01402. You will find this code most efficiently by reviewing the anesthesia section rather than the CPT Index. Find the knee header and review the codes. Total knee arthroplasty is the correct term for total knee replacement.

8. 00400, AA. Locate anesthesia, integumentary, leg. Both the upper and lower leg are specified, but they have the same code, which is for anesthesia services on the integumentary system. The question specified the procedure was performed by the anesthesiologist, which requires the AA modifier.

9. 00930, +99100. Locate anesthesia, orchiopexy in the CPT Index. The qualifying circumstance code is required to represent the patient's age.

10. 00921. Locate anesthesia, vasectomy in the CPT Index.

Multiple Choice

1. c

2. b

3. a

4. a. There was no neuraxial labor analgesia provided; therefore, neither 01967 nor 01968 can be reported.

5. d. 00400 is the "not otherwise specified" code and is correct because a breast biopsy has no specific anesthesia code. The CRNA's services must have both anesthesia modifiers representing the CRNA's work under the supervision of the anesthesiologist.

6. a. Placement of the central venous catheter does not imply an emergency procedure; therefore, 99140 would be incorrect.

7. b

8. c

9. b

10. d

Short Answer

1. Possible answers are preoperative visits, postoperative visits, administration of fluids or blood, and the usual monitoring services.

2. 00320–P4

3. 01630

4. 23, 47

5. Qualifying circumstances

6. That service would not be reported. Preoperative services are included in the anesthesia codes.

7. No, physical status modifiers are appended to anesthesia codes only.

8. 00567

9. 01382

10. No, 01968 is an add-on code that must be reported with code 01967.

Case Studies

1. 00940–AA. LEEP is an excision of tissue from the cervix as indicated in the procedure note. The correct code would be found under the perineum header in the anesthesia section or locate anesthesia, vagina in the CPT Index. The procedure note also specified the anesthesiologist provided the anesthesia and the –AA modifier would be appended.

2. 01482 –QZ. You will find this code most efficiently by reviewing the anesthesia section rather than the CPT Index. Find the lower leg header and review the codes. The procedure specified the services of CRNA and the –QZ modifier must be appended.

3. 00103 –QX, –QS. Locate anesthesia, eyelid in the CPT Index to find code 00103. The case study specified that you code for the CRNA; this requires the –QX modifier to indicate the CRNA was medically directed by the anesthesiologist because the presence of the anesthesiologist was in the procedure note. Correct coding also requires the –QS modifier for the monitored anesthesia care (MAC).

4. –23. When general anesthesia is provided for a procedure that normally would be done under a local anesthetic, append modifier –23, the "unusual anesthesia" modifier.

5. 00840, –P3, 99100, –AA, 3. You will find this code most efficiently by reviewing the anesthesia section rather than the CPT Index. Find the lower abdomen header; the appendix is considered intraperitoneal and you will report the not otherwise specified code 00840. The patient's uncontrolled diabetes requires the –P3 modifier; his age is represented with the qualifying circumstance code 99100, and –AA is reported to represent the personal service of the anesthesiologist. There were three increments of time.

6. 00170, –AA, –23. This code is found in the CPT Index under intraoral, or go to the head header and review the codes; this is a not otherwise specified code. The AA modifier is appended because the presence of the anesthesiologist is documented and modifier –23 is required because this type of procedure is normally performed under local anesthetic.

7. 00530, –QX for the CRNA, 00530, –QY for the anesthesiologist. Use the CPT Index for anesthesia, pacemaker to find this code. The CRNA was under the medical direction of the anesthesiologist, requiring both modifiers.

8. 00120, –P3, +99100. Under the head header, the only available code for the procedure is the not otherwise specified code 00120. Modifier –P3 is required for the patient's severe systemic diseases and the qualifying circumstance modifier is reported to reflect his age.

9. 00400, –QZ. This would be considered an integumentary procedure, not otherwise specified, and requires the modifier for a CRNA without medical direction by an anesthesiologist.

10. 00920. This code would be found under the perineum header for the male genitalia, not otherwise specified.

CHAPTER 16 CPT: Surgery Codes

Code It!

1. 30300. The removal of foreign body codes are generally found in the beginning of the surgery sections under the removal header, or use the CPT Index under removal, foreign body, nose.

2. 33681. Find septal defect in the cardiovascular section of the CPT.

3. 69205. The removal of foreign body codes are generally in the beginning of the surgery sections under the removal header, or use the CPT Index under removal, foreign body.

4. 69505–RT. The auditory section of the CPT is small and can easily be reviewed for mastoidectomy.

5. 38221. Review the bone marrow section of the cardiovascular system in the CPT.

6. 69631. The auditory section of the CPT is small and can easily be reviewed for tympanoplasty.

7. 38115. The spleen codes are in a small section after the cardiovascular system in the CPT.

8. 69930. This code is easily found in the last part of the auditory section or use the CPT Index to find cochlear device, implantation.

9. 55400. In the male genital system of the CPT, find vas deferens.

10. 59820. Review the CPT Index for abortion, missed, first trimester.

Multiple Choice

1. b. The additional 60 minutes required for the procedure with documentation to support the additional time meets the criteria for modifier –22.

2. c. If a surgeon treats a patient within the postoperative period for a condition unrelated to the surgery, modifier –24 is appended to the E/M visit code.

3. c. The code description that follows the semicolon is part of the parent code and is not included in the description of the indented codes.

4. b. A patient's diagnosis provides the medical necessity for the performance of a surgical procedure.

5. b. The unrelated procedure modifier is –79. If the procedure is related to the previous surgery, it may be –58 or –78, depending on the circumstances. Modifier –62 is the co-surgery modifier.

6. c. Modifier –57 is used to indicate that the E/M encounter encompassed the decision to provide major surgery and the E/M encounter occurred the day before or the day of the surgery.

7. d. When an E/M service is provided and it is separate and distinct from the procedure performed on that same day, report modifier –25 with the E/M code.

8. b. A designated separate procedure can be reported if it is the only procedure performed during that session. If performed with another, more major procedure, it is included in that more major procedure unless it is performed in a separate site or during a separate session on that same day.

9. a. Diagnostic procedures provide the information for a physician to determine what course of treatment is needed.

10. a. Modifier –47 signifies that the surgeon provided the anesthesia and the surgery. The surgeon would not report an anesthesia code; he or she would report the surgery code with modifier –47.

Short Answer

1. 12011–12018

2. 69610

3. New

4. 58555

5. 27447

6. 17000

7. 35201

8. 11604

9. 19318

10. 52204

Case Studies

1. No, modifier –52 is used only with procedure codes, not E/M codes.

2. Modifier –50, because breast codes are unilateral unless the code description states otherwise. The identical procedure was performed on both breasts and modifier 50 is the bilateral modifier.

3. Modifier –78, because this modifier is used to indicate that a return to the operating room was required because of a complication of a previous surgery.

4. The phrase "an incision was made, revealing the patella"

5. Thoracotomy, because if an incision is made into the chest area it is no longer wound repair.

6. No, modifier –51 is never reported with an add-on code.

7. No, the admission for further testing is not considered major surgery, which is the criteria for the use of modifier –57.

8. No, the exploratory laparotomy code is a designated separate procedure, which means that it cannot be reported when another more major procedure is performed at the same time at the same site.

9. Thoracotomy, because the "ostomy" suffix means there was a surgical creation of an opening for drainage.

10. Endoscopic, based on the term *arthroscopy* as indicated in the operation header; the left shoulder, as indicated in the operation header. The sutures were noted at the end of the operative report "#2 Orthocord and Krakow.

CHAPTER 17 CPT: Integumentary System

Code It!

1. 19301. As the CPT breast guidelines indicate, lumpectomy is considered a partial mastectomy procedure.

2. 11443. To correctly code for excisions, determine if the lesion is benign or malignant, choose the correct parent code based on anatomical location, and then find the correct dimension code.

3. 11307

4. 11901

5. 12020

6. 17313

7. 17000, 17003

8. 17250

9. 11200, 11201x2

10. 15734

Multiple Choice

1. b. The correct answer must have two codes, one for each excision. Answer a, code 11401, is in the wrong site, and answer d, code 11420–51, is in the wrong site.

2. c. The correct answer must have two codes because there were two different treatments provided, debridement and surgical repair, and they were performed in separate sites.

3. a. This was a simple repair. Answer b was intermediate, c was the incorrect site, and d was for an incorrect measurement.

4. d. All repairs were in the same parent code description and all were complex. To answer correctly, you would add all the repairs together and report accordingly.

5. a. The extensive undermining of tissue makes the layered (intermediate) closure complex. Answer d is in the wrong site.

6. c. The correct answer must have two codes, one for the preparation of the site and the second for the actual split-thickness graft.

7. d. The scar excision with repair by dorsal nasal flap is an adjacent tissue transfer (ATT) procedure. Only the ATT code is reportable; the scar excision is included in the ATT code.

8. b. Answer a is a full-thickness graft but for the incorrect site, c is a split-thickness graft, and d is for site preparation.

9. d. First select the correct parent code based on the anatomical site 17311. There was an additional stage performed requiring that add-on code 17312 be reported. Any answer with modifier –51 is incorrect. That modifier is never used with an add-on code.

10. b. Review the wound repair guidelines, specifically instruction #4. It directs you to the wound exploration guidelines for this procedure.

Short Answer

1. No, excision includes biopsy of the same lesion.

2. 12032. Combine the dimensions of the same classification repairs within the same anatomical site based on the code description.

3. 19296

4. Adjacent tissue transfer

5. 15100, 15101. Code 15100 represents the first 100 sq. cm, the add-on code 15101 is used for each additional 100 sq. cm or any part of the additional 100 sq. cm.

6. 11005

7. 17000, 17003x9. Code 17000 represents the first lesion, and add-on code 17003 represents each additional lesion after the first.

8. 17004. Once you have treated more than 14 lesions, you use code 17004 for 15 or more lesions.

9. 17311, 17315

10. One code, 19368, because 19368 incorporates all of 19367.

Case Studies

1. 19318–50. Key words are *reduction* and *bilateral*. Find the code by looking up "reduction" and then "breast." The procedure was accurately indicated in the header of the documentation and modifier –50 is needed to indicate the bilateral procedure.

2. 13131. Although the documentation indicates layered closure, which would be an intermediate repair, the scar revision portion of the repair makes the repair complex.

3. 11422, 13121–51. A nevus is a benign lesion; the closure was stated as complex. The excision code is the more major procedure and would be reported first.

4. 19020. Look up "exploration" of the "breast" in the CPT Index; the code description for 19020 indicates the drainage of abscess.

5. 11623. Basal cell carcinoma is a malignant lesion. The correct measurement of the lesion incorporates the 0.2 cm (2-mm) margin at each end of the diameter of the lesion, creating a 2.4 excision size.

6. 15830. An abdominoplasty is also referred to as a panniculectomy or lipectomy. In searching the CPT Index for abdominoplasty, it directs you to panniculectomy, which directs you to lipectomy.

7. 19325–50. Breast augmentation is found in the CPT Index under breast and augmentation. There are two codes based on whether or not implants are placed at the time of the procedure. The documentation indicates implants were placed. Modifier –50 is required because the procedure was bilateral.

8. 11770. Look in the CPT Index under excision/cyst/pilonidal for the code range. Although the indications for the excision seem extensive, the actual procedure documented is considered simple based on the type of closure.

9. 11406, 11406–51. Lipomas or fatty tumors are considered skin lesions unless they enter into the muscle area. Both excised lipomas were excised down to the subcutaneous layer and are coded as benign skin lesions. Both excised areas are within the same parent code description; therefore, modifier –51 is used to indicate multiple procedures.

10. 15100, +15101. Skin graft coding is based on the recipient site, which in this case is the right lower extremity, the same location as the donor site.

CHAPTER 18 CPT: Musculoskeletal System

Code It!

1. 25530

2. 28505 (do not code for the cast, because it is included)

3. 29881–RT

4. 23930–RT

5. 28080–LT

6. 29880–LT

7. 29075–LT

8. 25111

9. 27840

10. 27562

Multiple Choice

1. d. Two codes are required to report arthrodesis to L3–L5: Code 22612 for L3–L4, and add-on code 22614 for L4–L5.

2. c. This is a posterior nonsegmental instrumentation procedure. Answers a and b are segmental.

3. d. The correct answer requires two codes because both the cage placement and bone graft must be reported.

4. d. Answers a and c are incorrect because you cannot report a diagnostic arthroscopy (29870) with a surgical arthroscopy.

5. b. Review the notes in this code area.

6. d. The arthroscopic procedure will be included in the open procedure if both are performed on the same site.

7. c. A separate procedure may be reported if it is the only procedure performed or if performed in a separate site or during a separate session as another, more major procedure. When performed in a separate site or session, report modifier –59 on the separate procedure code.

8. a. Answer a represents the only possible correct answer.

9. a. The correct answer must have modifier –79 because these are two unrelated procedures; the tendon repair was performed during the global period of the ankle dislocation. The tendon repair is on the right foot, whereas the ankle is on the left.

10. b. Using the CPT Index, talectomy leads to astragalectomy and that is code 28130 under the foot and toes header. Using CPT or chapter illustrations, you will find the talus on the foot near the heel.

Short Answer

1. Yes, it is not included in the code description for 23670.

2. Modifier –59, because the wound exploration codes are separate procedures and would be included in another, more major procedure performed during the same operative session UNLESS it is in a separate site or performed during a separate session.

3. The coder, because the code is based on the number of muscles injected.

4. No, modifier –62 is never reported with bone grafts.

5. Yes, there is a parenthetical note under code 20955 indicating that the code should not be reported with code 69990.

6. No, to report code 21073 the manipulation must be performed under a general anesthetic.

7. No, discectomy is included in the arthrodesis code when it is performed in order to accomplish the arthrodesis.

8. No, the correct code is 21734.

9. No, the replacement cast can be reported.

10. 20692

Case Studies

1. Code 20610. Locate injection and then bursa in the CPT Index to find this code.

2. Code 20605. Locate injection and then joint and review the code range in the CPT Index to find this code.

3. Code 28090. The procedure does state ganglion cyst, but in the CPT Index there are only two codes for ganglion cyst and both are for the wrist. To find the code for the foot, the coder would go to the word *cyst* in the CPT Index and find foot. The code description does have the word *ganglion* indicated.

4. Code 29875. The documentation does indicate a diagnostic arthroscopy but the coder would only code for the synovectomy procedure. A surgical arthroscopy always includes a diagnostic arthroscopy. There are two synovectomy codes and the coder should report limited code because the synovectomy was for plica in one compartment.

5. Code 29881. This code represents medial or lateral meniscectomy and the documentation states the procedure was performed in the lateral compartment of the knee.

6. Code 29827. This is a surgical shoulder arthroscopy with rotator cuff repair. Look up arthroscopy, surgical, shoulder in the CPT Index.

7. Code 27096. To find this code, go to injection, sacroiliac in the CPT Index. The code is unilateral (left); therefore, modifier 50 would not be appended.

8. Code 28292. The hallux valgus or bunion codes start with code 28290 and the coder can simply follow the codes until he or she finds the McBride bunionectomy; alternatively, the coder can look up McBride procedure in the CPT Index.

9. Code 26418. Locate repair in the CPT Index, then finger, then tendon.

10. Code 27814. Locate fracture in the CPT Index, then ankle, then bimalleolar. Note that the code description includes internal fixation.

CHAPTER 19 CPT: Respiratory System

Code It!

1. 31276–50, 30140–51–50. The endoscopic sinus procedure and turbinate resection codes are both reportable and require the bilateral modifier –50. The turbinate code also requires modifier –51 (the multiple surgery modifier).

2. 31237. The debridement procedure is reportable because the endoscopic sinus surgery codes do not have a global period.

3. 31254, 31256–51

4. 31629–73. The –73 modifier represents a facility modifier when a procedure is discontinued before the administration of anesthesia.

5. 31641

6. 31255, 31287–51

7. 32554

8. 31640

9. 30906. CPT provides a subsequent hemorrhage control code for the posterior nasal passage.

10. 31624

Multiple Choice

1. b. Answer a is for vestibular stenosis and d is for dermatoplasty.

2. a. Answer b is for both anterior and posterior ethmoidectomy and c is for a diagnostic endoscope.

3. a. Answer b is with removal of tissue, which is not indicated in the question; c is a diagnostic sinusoscopy; and d is not maxillary.

4. a. Answers b and d have codes for a diagnostic bronchoscopy, which is incorrect, and code 32482 is a bilobectomy.

5. c. Answer a is anterior only, b is incorrect because there was no indication of a bilateral procedure, and d has the –22 modifier without any justification.

6. a. Two codes are offered in the answers and code 30110 is specifically for the office setting.

7. d. The correct answer must have modifier –50, which eliminates b and c. Answer a is a scope procedure.

8. b. *Esophago* is for the esophagus, *myo* is muscle, and *otomy* is incision.

9. c. Two codes are offered in the answers, code 31002 is for lavage, and the correct answer must have modifier –50.

10. b. Two codes are offered in the answers, and code 32098 is for biopsy by thoracotomy. The correct answer must have code 77002 for the fluoroscopic guidance.

Short Answer

1. Indirect, because a direct laryngoscopy views directly through the scope.

2. 31605

3. No, code 31622 is a diagnostic bronchoscopy and a separate procedure. Code 31629 is a surgical bronchoscopy, which includes a diagnostic bronchoscopy.

4. Yes, code 32550 is performed in a separate site from code 32554 and can be reported with modifier –59. See note under code 32550.

5. Because the code description specifies "lungs"

6. 32488, because this is a completion pneumonectomy.

7. 31201

8. 30115–50

9. The pleura

10. Ostium

Case Studies

1. 32100 represents an exploratory thoracotomy.

2. 32663 represents the use of a thoracoscope to remove a lobe of the lung.

3. 32096 represents a wedge resection biopsy.

4. 32505 represents a thoracotomy wedge resection in one lobe of the lung.

5. 31360 represents a total laryngectomy with radical neck dissection.

6. 31603 specifically represents an emergency transtracheal tracheostomy.

7. 30520 represents a nasal septoplasty procedure.

8. 31238 represents control of nasal hemorrhage (epistaxis).

9. 32400 represents a percutaneous needle biopsy of the pleura.

10. 30300 represents the removal of a foreign body from within the nose in the physician's office.

CHAPTER 20 CPT: Cardiovascular, Hemic, and Lymphatic Systems

Code It!

1. 33227. Only code 33227 is reported; revision of the site is included in removal and reinsertion of the single-chamber pacemaker generator.

2. 33224. If the patient already has the pacemaker system in place, report code 33224 when the left ventricular electrode is placed. Code +33225 is reported when the left ventricular electrode is placed at the same time as the insertion of the pacemaker system.

3. 33214. This is an upgrade of a single-chamber system to a dual-chamber system.

4. Assign 38745. In the lymphadenectomy section (38700–38780), carefully review the descriptions to determine the correct anatomical area, cervical versus axillary, and superficial versus complete.

5. 36420. In the venipuncture section (36400–36425), review the descriptions for age and specific references to cutdown.

6. 33011, 76930. The pericardiocentesis codes 33010 and 33011 are differentiated by designations of initial versus subsequent. The RSI code is specified in the parenthetical notes below each code.

7. +35390. Just as there is a reoperation code for coronary artery bypass grafts, carotid thromboendarterectomy procedures also have a reoperation code. Go to the CPT Index and look under "Reoperation." The carotid artery is listed there, but never code from the CPT Index—always check the code description and guidelines before assigning a code.

8. 33915. Refer to the CPT Index under "Embolectomy"—the pulmonary artery is listed there.

9. 38101. Spleen codes range from 38100–38200, and the splenectomy code range is 38100–38102. A partial splenectomy is coded with 38101.

10. 34703, To code for endograft aortic aneurysm repairs, determine the type of prosthesis. Code 34703 represents the aortic-uni-iliac endograft that represents the surgery required for an infrarenal aortic aneurysm involving a unilateral iliac artery. The code includes any RSI work performed.

Multiple Choice

1. d. The intraoperative angiography is included in the bypass graft; therefore, answers a and b are incorrect. Answer c is a vein bypass graft, whereas the question specifies an in-situ graft.

2. b. You cannot use modifier –51 with an add-on code; therefore, a and c are incorrect. Answer d has an in-situ graft code, whereas the question specifies a vein graft.

3. a. Answer b is a temporary pacemaker code, c is an epicardial code, and the use of modifier –62 in answer d is incorrect, because the question did not indicate that two surgeons were involved.

4. a. Answer b is for subsequent pericardiocentesis and answers c and d are incorrect because there is no documentation of E/M key components in the question.

5. c. Answers a and b are external cardiac tumor codes, and answer d is incorrect because of the use of code 33141 for revascularization, which was not specified in the question.

6. a. Answer b is for ICD placement, c represents the procedure without cardiopulmonary bypass, and d is for ablation and reconstruction.

7. b. Answer a is for a thromboendarterectomy, c represents a ruptured condition, and in d you cannot report both codes together because the pseudoaneurysm is either ruptured or not.

8. c. Answer a is a traumatic diaphragmatic hernia, b is a hernia resection code, and d is a neonatal hernia.

9. a. The surgical exposure code is unilateral and the correct answer must have modifier –50. Answers c and d include a code for the prosthesis, which is not documented in the question.

10. d. Answers a, b, and c are aortic valve, mitral valvotomy, and mitral valvuloplasty, respectively.

Short Answer

1. Yes, a single-chamber pulse generator has one attachment for the electrode. It must be replaced with a pulse generator that has two attachments.

2. 33249 is the standard code for insertion of a pacing cardioverter defibrillator.

3. 33512, do not report codes 33517–33523, which are add-on codes to be reported only with artery codes 33533–33536.

4. Use add-on code 35572.

5. In situ vein

6. The five vascular systems are venous, arterial, pulmonary, portal, and lymphatic.

7. Two, one for the artery and an add-on code for the vein portion of the combined vein and artery grafts.

8. The great vessels of the heart are the aorta, pulmonary artery, pulmonary veins, superior vena cava, and inferior vena cava.

9. Yes, review of the parent code description for 36221 shows that the RSI is included in this series of codes. The general guidelines for vascular injections indicate that nonselective catheterizations are included in selective catheterizations.

10. No, the parenthetical note under code 33256 indicates that you cannot report both codes; however, the guidelines for codes 33250–33261 indicate that add-on codes 33257–33259 are reported when both services are provided.

Case Studies

1. 34001. Locate embolectomy, then carotid in the CPT Index.

2. 35301. Locate endarterectomy in the CPT Index, which then refers you to thromboendarterectomy and carotid.

3. 33405. In coding for aortic valve replacements, you need to determine if it was performed transcatheter or as an open procedure. This operative report indicates it was an open procedure. Locate replacement, aortic valve, and review the codes indicated for the open procedure.

4. 37221. In coding for revascularization, you need to be aware of the coding hierarchy for these procedures. The operative report indicates that both balloon angioplasty and stenting were performed but you are allowed to code only for the stent, which includes the balloon angioplasty.

5. 35875. This operative report indicates that both thrombosis and intraoperative angiography were performed. Any intraoperative angiography is included in performing the procedure and cannot be reported separately. To code for the procedure, locate thrombectomy, then bypass graft (other than hemodialysis or fistula), and review the code range indicated.

6. 33510. For coronary bypass graft coding, you need to know which material was used for the graft and how many grafts were performed. The key identifiers in the operative report are "severe coronary disease," and "Saphenous vein was taken," and "We then bypassed the right coronary artery." Each of these indicates one artery was bypassed with a vein graft.

7. 37619. Locate ligation, vein, vena cava to find this code. It is also important to note that an additional procedure was performed but it is included in the ligation. Exploratory laparotomy is a designated separate procedure and is included in performing the ligation.

8. 35371. Locate endarterectomy in the CPT Index, which then refers you to thromboendarterectomy and common femoral. Intraoperative angiography is included in the performance of the thromboendarterectomy.

9. 33875. Descending thoracic aneurysm repairs can be repaired as endovascular or open procedures. The operative report does not indicate an endovascular repair.

10. 34701. The key to coding for endovascular abdominal aortic aneurysms is to find the correct prosthetic used for the repair. This repair used an aorto-aortic prosthesis. These codes start with 34701 and from there you can identify the correct prosthesis. To use the CPT Index, locate endovascular repair. The RSI work is included in the endograft repair.

CHAPTER 21 CPT: Digestive System

Code It!

1. 45320
2. 46257
3. 43194
4. 43264
5. 42700
6. 49572
7. 45910
8. 42107
9. 44147
10. 42405

Multiple Choice

1. c
2. a
3. d
4. d
5. b
6. a
7. a
8. d
9. a
10. a

Short Answer

1. 45378
2. 44186
3. 43214
4. 47600, 44950–52
5. 42106
6. 43754
7. 40510
8. Where, therapeutic, extent
9. 43255
10. 43845

Case Studies

1. 45384

2. a. 43239, 43757. b. Yes, by the anesthetist, not the surgeon.

3. G0121, Medicare requires HCPCS G codes for screening colonoscopy.

4. a. Dilation. b. Distal one third of esophagus. c. Duodenum. d. 43239, 43248–51.

5. a. Yes, ileocecal valve marks that scope reached the cecum. b. 43239, 45378–51.

6. a. No, patient had symptoms such as blood in the stool. b. 45378.

7. a. No, included in surgical package. b. No, included in surgical package. Because there is no documentation that this was performed for post-op pain control, it is included in procedural service. c. 46947.

8. 44388

9. 46275

10. 44382

CHAPTER 22 CPT: Urinary System

Code It!

1. 52240, 52283–51

2. 52325, 52332–51

3. 52270

4. 52005

5. 50590

6. 52318

7. 50200

8. 52320–RT

9. 50541

10. 52332

Multiple Choice

1. d

2. b

3. b

4. b

5. d

6. d

7. c

8. a

9. b

10. d

Short Answer

1. 50575–LT

2. 52234

3. 51990

4. 50323

5. 52000, 51727–51

6. 52341–50

7. 51702

8. 51798

9. 53440

10. 52318

Case Studies

1. 53020

2. 52000

3. 50590–RT

4. 52224

5. 52240, 52235–51

6. 52354–RT, 52354–RT–59. Code descriptor does not include the word *lesion(s)*, and because there were two tumors destroyed, the code is reported twice.

7. 52341–LT, 52332–51. CPT coding instructions say not to use 52351 in addition to 52341; however, 52351 is not an inherently bilateral code. CCI edit (facility and professional) indicates that 52351 is always part of 52341. Some insurers may allow 52351–RT–59 if they do not follow Medicare CCI logic.

8. 50590, 52310–51

9. 51880. In order to properly code this, you must know what a vesicostomy is and interchange with cystostomy.

10. 50693, 50390–59

CHAPTER 23 CPT: Male Genital System

Code It!

1. 54650

2. 55250

3. 55040

4. 54163

5. 54520

6. 55700

7. 55873

8. 52630

9. 54205

10. 54400

Multiple Choice

1. b

2. d

3. c

4. d

5. c

6. b

7. a

8. c

9. d

10. c

Short Answer

1. 55400–50, 69990

2. 54161

3. 11422. There is only one scrotum and the code descriptor has multiple body parts included so no LT modifier applies.

4. 54840–RT, 55060–50

5. 55705

6. 55110, 54840–LT–51

7. 10060

8. 54692–RT, 49650–RT–51

9. 54520–50

10. 54600–LT

Case Studies

1. 54161

2. 55520-LT

3. 54336. In this case, you need to determine what kind of hypospadias is being corrected. Subcoronal hypospadias is distal and perineal.

4. 54300

5. 54163

6. 55700, 76942–26

7. 55250

8. 54692-LT. The testis was in the abdomen; therefore, it required laparoscopy.

9. 54400. No modifier is required because the penis is not a paired body organ. Prosthesis is semi-rigid and there is no mention of it being multicomponent or inflatable.

10. a. No, it was only a temporary catheter and removed at the end of the procedure. b. 54640–RT–22, 49320. Laparoscopy was a diagnostic lap to assess the status and condition of both testes and is separately reported. The orchiopexy is a repeat procedure and extensive scar tissue had to be resected to free the testes and vas. The –22 modifier is also reported.

CHAPTER 24 CPT: Female Genital System and Maternity Care and Delivery

Code It!

1. 57461
2. 56740
3. 58672
4. 58350
5. 59812
6. 59320
7. 58545
8. 58555
9. 59841
10. G0101

Multiple Choice

1. b
2. a
3. c
4. a
5. b
6. c
7. a
8. b
9. b
10. d

Short Answer

1. 59160
2. 59410, 59412–51
3. 57110
4. 59841
5. 57106
6. 56620. 56810 cannot be reported separately because it is bundled according to CCI with no modifier override.

7. Anesthesiologist: 01960; OB/GYN: 59400, 59070–26

8. 59812

9. 59400

10. 59510, 58611

Case Studies

1. 58558

2. 58671

3. 57513

4. a. True. b. False. c. 58662, 58563–51.

5. 57135

6. 59820

7. 58561

8. a. 59400. b. 59514–59.

9. 58670

10. 56700

CHAPTER 25 CPT: Endocrine and Nervous Systems

Code It!

1. 64755

2. 64836, 64837, 69990

3. 63650

4. 60200

5. 61210

6. 61519

7. 60210

8. 61697

9. 64795

10. 62272

Multiple Choice

1. c

2. b

3. d

4. a

5. b

6. b

7. c

8. a

9. c

10. a

Short Answer

1. 61514

2. No, code 60540 is included in the kidney removal (nephrectomy) codes. The code description for 60540 states "(separate procedure)" which means 60540 can be reported if it is the only procedure being performed. If performed with another procedure, it is included in the other procedure unless 60540 is performed in a separate site or during a separate session that day. Because the adrenal gland sits on top of the kidney, its removal would be included in the nephrectomy.

3. 63081. The corpectomy is when part or all of the actual vertebral body is removed. The discectomy is when the cartilage cushion between the vertebrae (disk) is removed. If he removes 30% to 50% or more of the vertebral body, the corpectomy code is reported. The code is only reported once because it consists of one segment.

4. 62287. Category III code 0274T doesn't work because no laminotomy or laminectomy was performed. Fluoro is bundled into this procedure.

5. 61850

6. 63075

7. a. Lumbar. b. Laminectomy. c. One. d. 63030.

8. a. Therapeutic. b. Epidural space or spine. c. What. d. Approach. e. Continuous. f. Bilateral. h. Interspace (for spine injections) or nerve injections.

9. 64721–RT, 64727

10. 64831–F8, 64872, 69990. The patient did not see the orthopedist for 4 days with surgery 5 days post injury.

Case Studies

1. 64895, 69990

2. 64600

3. 62258, 62160

4. 63650

5. 64718–RT

6. 64483–RT, 64484–RT

7. 64493–50, 64494–50, 64495–50

8. 64490–50

9. 63030–LT, 69990

10. 64405–50, 64450 x 2. The greater occipital nerve originates from the medial branch of the dorsal portion of the C2 spinal nerve and provides sensory innervation to the midline back of the scalp area. Report with 64405 for each side. In contrast, the lesser occipital nerve originates from the lateral branch of the ventral portion of the C2 and sometimes the C3 spinal nerve. It provides sensory innervation to the lateral scalp area behind the ear. Report with 64450 once for each aide as there isn't a specific code for lesser occipital nerve injection.

CHAPTER 26 CPT: Eye and Ear

Code It!

1. 69436–50

2. 67825–E3

3. 69610, 69990

4. 66986–LT

5. 69433–LT

6. 68200–LT

7. 68801–RT

8. 67938–E1, 14060–51

9. 69200–RT

10. 12011

Multiple Choice

1. d

2. c

3. b

4. c

5. d

6. b

7. a

8. d

9. d

10. b

Short Answer

1. 69661–RT. L8615 is the HCPCS code for the implant; however, you may not have learned to code that yet.

2. 69210–RT

3. 68420–LT

4. Tympanostomy refers to the surgical procedure. Myringotomy is a surgical technique. Tympanic ventilation is the purpose or outcome of the procedure.

5. 65286–LT

6. Any of the following are correct answers. (a) How many muscles are involved; (b) which muscles are involved, by name, so codes can be assigned according to medial, lateral, or superior oblique muscle; (c) if the patient had strabismus surgery previously; (d) if a patient had surgery on the eye previously not involving extraocular muscles; (e) if adjustable sutures are placed; (f) if posterior fixation sutures are placed; (g) if transposition of extra-ocular muscles is performed.

7. CPT provides instruction either preceding or following both codes regarding which proce-dures may be reported with each. 66990. Use of ophthalmic endoscope may be used only with codes 65820, 65875, 65920, 66985, 66986, 67036, 67039, 67040, 67041, 67042,

67043, 67112, and 67113. This scope is used only for procedures on the eye where the probe tip is inserted through sclerotomy. It is necessary to use when there are pathological changes or failure of the pupil to dilate. CPT 69990 is a surgical microscope, not an endoscope, and is used for procedures performed in all body systems.

8. 67040–RT

9. Trabeculectomy. Trabeculoplasty is performed with a laser using heat to shrink the trabecular mesh and pulling open the areas not treated to allow aqueous to drain. No incisions are made and no tissue is removed. During a trabeculectomy, a microscope is used and a flap is created.

10. The following are indications that a complex cataract extraction with IOL placement was performed (66982). Most cataracts performed in the pediatric age group qualify. Pediatric anatomy contributes to the complexity of cataract surgery. The anterior capsule tears with great difficulty and the cortex is difficult to remove from the eye because of intrinsic adhesion of the lens material. Additionally, a primary posterior capsulotomy or capsulorrhexis is necessary, which further complicates the insertion of the intraocular lens. Patients who present with diseased states, prior intraocular surgery, or with dense, hard, or white cataracts also qualify. The presence of trauma, or weak or abnormal lens support structures caused by numerous conditions (e.g., uveitis) and disease states (e.g., glaucoma, pseudoexfoliation syndrome, Marfan syndrome), require additional surgical involvement, as well as utilization of additional techniques and surgical devices. A small pupil found in a patient with glaucoma or a past surgical history may cause the eye to not dilate fully, requiring iris retractors through additional incisions. Capsular support rings to allow the placement of an intraocular lens may be required in the presence of weak or absent support structures. Medicare contractors have information regarding documenting complex cataracts on their websites.

Case Studies

1. 65850–RT

2. 65755–RT, V2785

3. 66984–LT

4. 67801–E3

5. 65426–RT

6. 69620–RT, 21235

7. 69436–RT, 92502–59–LT

8. 69632–LT, 15770

9. 67311–50

10. 67923–E4

CHAPTER 27 CPT: Radiology Codes

Code It!

1. 73070–LT

2. 78013

3. 76705

4. 77299

5. 76604

6. 77290

7. 71046, 76000

8. 77067

9. 70460–TC

10. 73521, 72170–51

Multiple Choice

1. a

2. c

3. b

4. d

5. d

6. c

7. c

8. d

9. b

10. a

Short Answer

1. a. A-mode refers to a one-dimensional ultrasonic measurement procedure. M-mode refers to a one-dimensional ultrasonic measurement procedure with movement of the trace to record amplitude and velocity of moving echo-producing structures.

   b. B-scan refers to a two-dimensional ultrasonic scanning procedure with a two-dimensional display Real-time scan refers to a two-dimensional ultrasonic scanning procedure with display of both two-dimensional structure and motion with time.

2. 77080

3. a. 77078, 77079, 77080, 77081, 77083, 76977, or G0130 (HCPCS). Technically, there isn't a code specifically designated for "screening" DEXA, but these are the ones that are recognized by the payer. b. 77080. c. Sources: IOM-100-04 Chapter 13 Section 140, Transmittal 1416 01-18-2008 CR 5847, LCDs, Article A51974. Coverage policies are consistent for screening DEXA, indicating it is not a covered service. "Bone density measurement is not a covered Medicare benefit when utilized for osteoporosis screening in an estrogen-deficient woman, who <u>has not been</u> determined by the physician or a qualified non-physician practitioner treating her to be at clinical risk for osteoporosis, based on her medical history and other findings." DEXA is performed on a qualified individual (patient) for the purpose of identifying bone mass, detecting bone loss, or determining bone quality. Patients must meet at least one of the five following criteria for a DEXA to be covered.

   - A woman who has been determined by the physician or a qualified nonphysician practitioner treating her to be estrogen-deficient and at clinical risk for osteoporosis, based on her medical history and other findings (reason to do screening)
   - An individual receiving (or expecting to receive) glucocorticoid (steroid) therapy equivalent to 5 mg of prednisone, or greater, per day, for more than three (3) months (screening)
   - An individual with primary hyperparathyroidism (screening)
   - An individual with vertebral abnormalities as demonstrated by an x-ray to be indicative of osteoporosis, osteopenia (low BONE mass), or vertebral fracture (diagnostic or monitoring DEXA)
   - An individual being monitored to assess the response to or efficacy of an FDA-approved osteoporosis drug therapy (monitoring)

- Contractors will pay claims for monitoring tests when billed with CPT 77080 and diagnosis of osteoporosis, disorder of bone and cartilage, or Cushing syndrome.

4. a. An official interpretation (final report) by the interpreting physician must be generated and archived following any examination, procedure, or officially requested consultation regardless of the site of performance (hospital, imaging center, physician office, mobile unit, etc.). It is not appropriate for nonphysicians to provide interpretations or generate diagnostic reports (final or preliminary).

   b. Components of the Report

   1. **Demographics**

      a. The facility or location where the study was performed

      b. Name of patient and another identifier

      c. Patient's date of birth or age

      d. Patient's gender

      e. Name(s) of ordering physician(s) or other health-care provider(s)

   2. **Name or type of examination**

   3. **Date of the examination**

      Time of the examination, if relevant (e.g., for patients who are likely to have more than one of a given examination per day)

   4. **Relevant clinical information**

   5. **Procedures and materials**

      The report should include a description of the studies or procedures performed and any contrast media or radiopharmaceuticals (including specific administered activities, concentration, volume, and route of administration when applicable), medications, catheters, or devices used, if not recorded elsewhere. Any known significant patient reaction or complication should be recorded.

   6. **Findings**

      The report should use appropriate anatomical, pathological, and radiological terminology to describe the findings.

   7. **Potential limitations**

      If any, identify factors that may compromise the sensitivity and specificity of the examination, as well as any unforeseen circumstances, complications, or patient reactions.

   8. **Comparison studies and reports**

      If applicable and appropriate, comparison with relevant examinations and reports should be part of the radiological consultation and report.

   9. **Impression (conclusion or diagnosis)**

      A specific diagnosis should be given when possible. A differential diagnosis should be entered when appropriate. Follow-up or additional diagnostic studies to clarify or confirm the impression should be suggested when appropriate.

5. If you are the coder assigning procedure and diagnosis codes for the radiologist, you are permitted to use the radiology reports. Coding directly from radiology reports is prohibited for inpatient coders. *Coding Clinic* addresses this topic, as does AHIMA and other sources focusing on compliance. Abnormal findings (laboratory, x-ray, pathological, and other diagnostic results) are not coded and reported unless the attending or consulting physician indicates their clinical significance. The radiology reports are used to obtain information such as laterality, if dye was used, and to obtain specificity for diagnosis coding once the physician has

noted the significance of the impression from the radiology service. For example, if a physician documents that a patient has a hip fracture, the coder can utilize the x-ray report that shows that there is a fracture of the lesser trochanter to assign a more specific diagnosis. This is allowable because the physician originally acknowledged a hip fracture, and the x-ray simply identified the specific location of the fracture.

6. The answer is located within the Radiology guidelines and E/M guidelines. When imaging is not included in the surgical procedure code or procedure from the medicine section of CPT, image guidance codes, those that state "radiological supervision and interpretation," may be reported for the imaging service.

   Written report(s)
   - A written report, signed by the interpreting physician, should be considered an integral part of a radiological procedure or interpretation.

   - The E/M documentation guidelines also address the need for a separate written report if the physician is reporting the professional interpretation of x-rays, as follows:

   "The actual performance and/or interpretation of diagnostic tests/studies ordered during a patient encounter are not included in the levels of E/M services. Physician performance of diagnostic tests/studies for which specific CPT codes are available may be reported separately, in addition to the appropriate E/M code. The physician's interpretation of the results of diagnostic tests/studies (i.e., professional component) with preparation of a separate distinctly identifiable signed written report may also be reported separately, using the appropriate CPT code with modifier 26 appended."

7. The **ordering** physician's order dictates the intent of the service. If the referring or ordering physician requests a screening mammography, that is the study that is performed and reported. However, if there are any abnormalities found on the screening images, the radiologist can either immediately perform a diagnostic mammogram or request the patient return to the imaging center for the diagnostic study without having to obtain an additional order from the referring physician.

8. The number of views and specific views obtained both play a role in code assignment. Radiology codes are chosen based on the number of views. Being able to identify the specific views enables a coder to count the number of views taken and select the correct code. Code descriptions include verbiage such as "minimum of two views" or "complete."

9. 70100 or 70110 cannot be reported bilaterally. Code description says "mandible." Mandible is not a paired body part.

10. The Medicare Physician Relative Value Guide or the Medicare Physician Fee Schedule (MPFS) has columns designated for PC/TC to signify when a code can be billed globally, or with –TC or –26 modifiers. It also contains a bilateral column with an indicator for each code, whether or not a code may be reported bilaterally.

Case Studies

1. 77785–TC

2. a. 74018–26. b. 74018–TC.

3. a. 72193–26. b. 72193–TC.

4. a. 23350–LT. b. 23350–LT. No –26 or –TC modifiers are appropriate for this service.

5. a. 73040–26–LT. b. 73040–TC–LT.

6. a. 73222–26. b. 73222–TC.

7. 78306

8. 76770. The procedure is performed in a physician's office; the physician owns the equipment and interprets the images.

9. a. 77778–26, 77290–26, 76965–26. b. 77778–TC, 77290–TC, 76965–TC. c. HCPCS code for seed sources.

10. a. 70200–26, 73050–LT–26. b. 70200–TC, 73050–LT–TC.

CHAPTER 28 CPT: Pathology and Laboratory Codes

Code It!

1. 82803

2. 88304

3. 80055

4. 81015

5. 84403

6. 82565

7. 89320

8. 85060

9. 82106

10. 88309

Multiple Choice

1. b

2. d

3. a

4. a

5. b

6. c

7. b

8. d

9. c

10. a

Short Answer

1. Presence

2. Six

3. Whether the surgeon, treating physician, or the pathologist indicates in the final report that separately identifiable analysis was required and documented by a final diagnosis.

4. FOBT is an abbreviation for fecal occult blood test. This is considered a colorectal cancer screening service. Code 82270 is used for non-Medicare patients. Medicare requires HCPCS code G0328 for FOBT, which is paid under the clinical diagnostic laboratory fee schedule. FOBTs may be paid for beneficiaries who have attained age 50, and at a frequency of once every 12 months. FOBT is typically guaiac-based, which tests for peroxidase activity. The beneficiary completes it by taking samples from two different sites of three consecutive stools. This screening requires a written order from the beneficiary's

attending physician. G0328 Screening FOBT, immunoassay, includes the use of a spatula to collect the appropriate number of samples or the use of a special brush for the collection of samples, as determined by the individual manufacturer's instructions. This screening requires a written order from the beneficiary's attending physician.

5. 88141, 88307

6. Office: 36415, 36416, 85018; Lab: 82607

7. 88307, 99360

8. G0431, G0434, and G6030, as well as G6058 as appropriate.

9. Physician order and a diagnosis or reason for performing the test

10. A physician order or laboratory requisition form is required to accompany a specimen to the laboratory for any testing from the CLFS. All specimens must be accompanied by a diagnosis code from the treating or ordering physician and reason for performing the said tests. The laboratory must be able to determine if the intent of the requested test is for "screening" or "diagnostic" purposes as rules for reporting diagnoses are based upon this. CMS requires that claims for screening tests located on the CLFS contain the same diagnosis submitted by the treating physician regardless of the outcome of testing. They must assign the submitted diagnostic information that was provided by the treating physician in ALL instances. In this case, laboratory and pathology coders cannot code directly from the laboratory report. If a laboratory test was ordered as a diagnostic test and the laboratory test was interpreted by the pathologist, then it is appropriate to assign the pathologist's interpretation of the laboratory test ONLY if those results are more definitive than the submitted diagnostic information by the ordering physician. Diagnoses for tests located on the MPFS are based upon what the ordering physician provided at the time the service was ordered. The laboratory or pathologist must report the diagnostic code provided by the ordering or referring physician. If no code is provided, laboratory tests are permitted to assign a diagnosis based upon the diagnostic statement or narrative provided with the test requisition.

Case Studies

1. 80305. Read the notes at the beginning of the *Guidelines* section. It explains that 80305–80307 are used for all drugs and drug classes. Alcohol and Ecstasy are both Class A. The *Guidelines* state that this is reported once per day. There was no mention of chromatography or immunoassay. In this case, there were two drugs to confirm, so 80320 and 80359 are also reported.

2. 80200

3. 87116, 87206

4. 86950, 86904

5. 88305

6. 88305

7. a. 3. b. Two, the frozen sections came as two separate cassettes from different areas (anterior and posterior). c. No, comment meant that the frozen sections were performed intraoperatively and the surgeon was waiting to hear that margins were clear before ending the procedure. The pathologist was not requested to be in the OR. d. 88305 x 3, 88331, 88331–59.

8. 88304

9. 88307

10. 88329, 88300. No microscopic examination was performed.

CHAPTER 29 CPT: Medicine Codes

Code It!

1. 96372, 90378. As the guidelines indicate in the immunoglobulin range of codes, correct coding requires two codes: one for the administration and one for the immunoglobulin product itself. The correct administration codes are in the 96365–96368, 96372, 96374, 96375 series of codes.

2. 90471, 90658. Vaccinations also require two codes, one for the administration and one for the product. No counseling was indicated in the exercise; therefore, 90471 is correct. There are many flu vaccine codes so special attention must be given to the code descriptions. Code 90658 is correct.

3. 99050. The special services codes start with code 99000. Code 99050 specifies "at times other than regularly scheduled office hours."

4. 99175. This code is listed under the other services and procedures section starting with code 99170. To report this service, coders can go to the CPT Index under ipecac administration.

5. 90396, 96372. Code 90396 represents the immune globulin product, and code 96372 is the intramuscular administration code.

6. 96406. Codes 96401–96549 represent chemotherapy administration. Code 96406 is part of the injection and intravenous infusion range 96401–96417 and is reported for more than seven lesions injected.

7. 90961. The ESRD codes are based on per-month codes or per-day codes. They are age based and must specify the number of physician visits. The exercise specified the services were for a full month, the patient was 55 years old, and there were three face-to-face physician visits during the month.

8. 90924. Coders need to understand the global surgical package, which includes postoperative services in the surgery payment. CPT provides code 99024 to show that a postoperative visit was provided but no charge is put into the billing system. Code 99024 is part of the special services codes starting with code 99000.

9. 93025. This procedure is part of the cardiography series of services, codes 93000–93042. The CPT Index does not provide a reference, unfortunately.

10. 92977. There are two coronary thrombolysis codes: 92975 and 92977. They are differentiated by whether the administration is via intracoronary infusion or intravenous infusion.

Multiple Choice

1. a. Answers b, c, and d represent either an E/M service or an incorrect dosage amount and are incorrect. An IM injection of a therapeutic drug is part of the 96365–96379 range of codes.

2. b. The correct answer must have a code from the cardiac catheterization section that incorporates coronary angiography and an additional code for the thrombolysis. The correct answer also requires a modifier –26 on the cath code and modifier –51 on the thrombolysis code.

3. b. The correct answer would have both an administration code without counseling and the code for the hepatitis vaccine product. Answer a is incorrect, because there is no medical necessity for the 99211 code, and 90645 represents the influenza vaccine. Answer c does not have an administration code, and d is incorrect because there is no documentation of a history, examination, or medical decision making, which are required to report an E/M code.

4. b. Answer a is incorrect, because the injection service is not coded. Answer c is incorrect, because code 96360 is never reported times two; if additional time is spent, then the add-on code 96361 is reported. Answer d is incorrect, because code 96365 is for an infusion, not an IV push.

5. d. This question describes an echocardiogram. An electrocardiogram does not provide this type of information; a ventriculogram provides only an image of the blood flow through the heart ventricle(s), and an electroencephalogram is an angiography of the brain.

6. a. Because there is an existing appointment slot for emergencies, the physician can report only the E/M code. Code 99058 is used when the emergency disrupts the other scheduled office services. Code 99060 is incorrect, because it specifies "out of the office." Answer d is incorrect, because modifier –22 is not used with E/M services; it is for procedures only.

7. d. Answer d is correct, because the question specified external cardioversion. Answer a is incorrect, because there is no documentation of an ICD evaluation. Answer b is incorrect, because it specifies an internal cardioversion. Answer c is incorrect, because there was not an insertion of a temporary pacemaker.

8. c. This is an example of the per-day ESRD coding. The patient was in the hospital for 4 days, there was no complete assessment during the month, and the patient's age is 49 years. Answer a is incorrect, because it is a per-month code for a 12- to 19-year-old patient with four or more face-to-face physician visits. Answer b is incorrect, because it is a per-month code with four face-to-face physician visits, but the age range is correct for this patient. Answer d is incorrect, because it is for patients 2 years of age or younger.

9. a. There are specific chemotherapy codes in the range of 96440–96549 described as other injection and infusion services, and they include other services in the code description that would be used to provide this type of chemotherapy. Answer b is incorrect, because it is injected via a subcutaneous reservoir. Answer c is incorrect, because it is intra-arterial, and answer d is incorrect, because it covers subcutaneous or intramuscular issues, not subarachnoid issues.

10. b. Answer a is incorrect because the patient is older than 5 years. Answer c is incorrect because moderate sedation is billable service and d is incorrect because it is an add-on code to 99151 and 99152.

Short Answer

1. Only if another separately identifiable service above and beyond the allergy service (typically something unrelated, such as an illness) is provided during the same visit.

2. Modifier –50

3. 92551

4. 96372

5. 96372, 90375

6. 92004, 92015. The ophthalmology general services codes are divided by intermediate versus comprehensive. If an examination is done of the complete visual system, then the code is comprehensive. Determination of the refractive state is not included in the general services codes; therefore, code 92015 is also reported.

7. 97597

8. 93318

9. 96365

10. 95115

Case Studies

1. 90471, 90472, 90717, 90691, 92950. Codes 90471 and 90472 represent the administration of the two vaccines. Code 90717 represents the yellow fever vaccine product, and 90691 is the typhoid vaccine product. CPR is appropriately coded with 92950.

2. 90970 x 23. The ESRD codes are based on per-month codes or per-day codes. They are age based and must specify the number of physician visits. When the per-month services are

interrupted by hospitalization or vacation, the performance of a complete assessment during that month determines whether or not the coder will report the per-month code or the per-day code. This patient was on vacation that month for 7 days and a complete assessment was not performed. The per-day service is reported for 30 days less the 7 days on vacation. (The per-month codes are always based on a 30-day month.)

3. 93016. In many coding exercises, particularly in the test environment, more detail is provided than is needed to code the service. Part of the test strategy for coders is to be able to filter out what is not necessary. In the stress test codes 93015–93018, the correct answer is based on whether the physician provided both the professional and technical components or just the professional or the technical component with some variations. The stress test codes are appropriate for either exercise or pharmacological testing. In this exercise, the relevant information is that a stress test was ordered and provided but the physician only supervised the stress test (professional component) without interpretation or report. The correct answer is therefore 93016. Keep in mind that the additional information provided is very relevant clinically.

4. 92928, +92929, +92921. These intervention services use a hierarchy of coding that includes any lesser interventions when a stent is inserted. The two branches of the left anterior descending artery are represented by 92928 and add-on code 92929. Because the intervention in the right coronary artery was an angioplasty only, that service is reported with the add-on code 92921.

5. 93455. Catheter placement into the coronary arteries is part of the cardiac catheterization codes 93451–93533. The coronary angiography parent code is 93544. If the catheter is placed into a bypass graft only, the correct code is 93455. The cardiac catheterization codes include the imaging supervision and interpretation.

6. 92975. This is a thrombolysis procedure. To find the code, go to the CPT Index under thrombolysis and then coronary. You are given code 92975–92977. Code 92977 is intravenous; this procedure was intracoronary.

7. 93886–26. Provision of supervision and interpretation but not performance of the Doppler study and not having ownership of the equipment necessary to perform the study requires that modifier –26 be appended to the Doppler code. To find the correct Doppler code, go to the CPT Index under Doppler scan and look for intracranial arteries, then complete study.

8. 99050. The Medicine section of CPT incorporates special services codes that are adjuncts to the basic service provided. Services provided in the office at times other than the regularly scheduled office hours are reported with code 99050.

9. 96413, +96368. To correctly code for the hydration, prophylactic, and diagnostic injections and infusions in addition to chemotherapy, you must first identify the initial service that is the reason for the patient encounter. In this case, it is chemotherapy, and that is the primary code. Additionally, this patient required concurrent (at the same time) infusion of an antiemetic. In reviewing the codes that start with 96365, you need to identify the add-on code representing a concurrent service.

10. 90839. The psychotherapy guidelines provide codes related to a crisis either as an urgent scenario or for a history of crisis state. That code range is 90839–90840. The codes are time based, with code 90839 for the first 60 minutes.

CHAPTER 30 HCPCS

Code It!

1. L8610

2. L8659

3. S2300–LT

4. S2112

5. A4336

6. L8680 x 4

7. J1160

8. E0619

9. L6709

10. A4930

Multiple Choice

1. c

2. c

3. a

4. d

5. d

6. b

7. d

8. c

9. a

10. d

Short Answer

1. Quantity alert. Carrier discretion. Item packaged into APC rates.

2. Special coverage instructions. OPPS status. B not recognized by OPPS when submitted on Part B bill type.

3. Quantity alert. Special coverage. Use for Streptase. Instructions. OPPS status N. Packaged into APC rate. No separate payment made.

4. J2060. Code is N1 status, meaning it is packaged into an APC payment and no separate payment is made. Six units.

5. Knowing a patient's insurance (primary and secondary) plays an important role in procedure code assignment. Medicare in particular requires the use of HCPCS G codes for procedural services in lieu of a CPT code when one is available. Coders need to be aware of payer policies for which HCPCS codes are accepted and their expected use. J codes are universally reported for drugs. Medicaid often requires use of HCPCS S and T codes, which take precedence over CPT codes when available. Modifier assignment will also vary; if a patient has Medicare, the provider should know not to report modifier –59 and that Medicare has requirements for HCPCS modifiers to use instead.

6. Competitive Acquisition Program (CAP) Fee schedule

7. AU—Item furnished in conjunction with a urological, ostomy, or tracheostomy supply. This modifier identifies items that are eligible for reimbursement under multiple benefit or payment categories. AU is an abbreviation that means "each ear." It is used in ENT records and on orders for otic drops. At this time, the only codes with which this modifier may be used are:
   - A4217–Sterile water/saline, 500 mL
   - A4450—Tape, nonwaterproof, per 18 sq. in.
   - A4452—Tape, waterproof, per 18 sq. in.

- A5120—Skin barrier, wipes or swabs, each
- A6531—Gradient compression stocking, below knee, 30–40 mm Hg, each
- A6532—Gradient compression stocking, below knee, 40–50 mm Hg, each
- A6545—Gradient compression stocking, wrap, nonelastic, below knee, 30–50 mm Hg, each

8. J3490, S0189. Carriers do not cover this service and consider it experimental and investigational. Subcutaneous hormone pellet implantation of estrogen alone, or estrogen combined with testosterone, or testosterone alone when used as hormone replacement therapy for menopause, is considered investigational. See https://www.cms.gov/medicare-coverage-database/.

9. E0431. The code describes a portable gaseous oxygen system, rental; includes portable container, regulator, flowmeter, humidifier, cannula or mask, and tubing. This code is considered to be DME equipment. The code is highlighted blue in the HCPCS manual, indicating that there are special coverage instructions associated with this code. The source listed beneath this code is MED: 100-4, 20, 30.6. This is the IOM 100-04, Chapter 20, Section 30.6, which discusses oxygen rental and requires the use of the –RR modifier.

10. E0260. MED: 100-4, 23, 60.3. This is the IOM 100-04, Chapter 23, Section 60.3. It explains that a hospital bed must be billed with modifier KX, GA, or GZ to indicate whether or not coverage criteria have been met.

Case Studies

1. A4425

2. C1776

3. C1779 x 2 leads, C1785

4. Q4038

5. C1875

6. J2175

7. J3490

8. G0127

9. E0601

10. J1885